Understanding Child Abuse

The partners of child sex offenders tell their stories

Terry Philpot

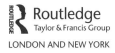

Routledge
Taylor & Francis Group

LONDON AND NEW YORK

First published 2009
by Routledge
2 Park Square, Milton Park, Abingdon, Oxon OX14 4RN

Simultaneously published in the USA and Canada
by Routledge
270 Madison Avenue, New York, NY 10016

Routledge is an imprint of the Taylor & Francis Group, an informa business

© 2009 Terry Philpot

Typeset in Sabon by
Taylor & Francis Books
Printed and bound in Great Britain by
TJ International Ltd, Padstow, Cornwall

All rights reserved. No part of this book may be reprinted or reproduced or
utilised in any form or by any electronic, mechanical, or other means, now
known or hereafter invented, including photocopying and recording, or in
any information storage or retrieval system, without permission in writing
from the publishers.

British Library Cataloguing in Publication Data
A catalogue record for this book is available from the British Library

Library of Congress Cataloging in Publication Data
Philpot, Terry.
   Understanding child abuse : the partners of child sex offenders tell their
stories / Terry Philpot.
      p. cm.
   1. Child sexual abuse–Case studies. 2. Child molesters–Family
relationships–Case studies. I. Title.
   HV6570.P495 2009
   362.76'3–dc22
   2008029207

ISBN 10: 0-415-40949-7 (hbk)
ISBN 10: 0-415-45600-2 (pbk)
ISBN 10: 0-203-88400-0 (ebk)

ISBN 13: 978-0-415-40949-0 (hbk)
ISBN 13: 978-0-415-45600-5 (pbk)
ISBN 13: 978-0-203-88400-3 (ebk)

Understanding Child Abuse

Understanding Child Abuse is the first book to look at women whose partners are child sex offenders. Much of the book is devoted to the voices of the women themselves, telling their stories and how they feel about the situations in which they found themselves, how they coped, and how they remade their lives and those of their families. They describe what they learned from their experience and how it changed them.

Such experience is largely overlooked by researchers, agencies and policy makers and this book throws unique light on this neglected area. The chapters cover:

- What we know about child sexual abuse, offenders and the effect of sexual abuse on children.
- A detailed description of the work which allows the women to explore and compare their experiences and feelings about what has happened.
- Verbatim interviews with both partners and offenders.

Combining theory, practice and personal testimony in a concise and accessible manner, *Understanding Child Abuse* is essential reading for social work practitioners and students as well as probation officers and anyone involved with child protection. It will also be of interest to members of the public.

Terry Philpot is the author and editor of more than a dozen books, including *Adoption* (with Anthony Douglas) and five books on working with sexually abused children. He is a trustee of the Social Care Institute for Excellence and of the Michael Sieff Foundation. He has won several awards for his journalism.

For Eddie Munting (1944–2008)
whose family was his life

Contents

The Men's Stories

About the author

Terry Philpot is a journalist and writer and a contributor to a wide range of publications. He has written and edited more than a dozen books, including (with Anthony Douglas) *Adoption: Changing Families, Changing Times* (Routledge, 2002); (with Julia Feast) *Searching Questions: Identity, Origins and Adoption* (BAAF, 2003); (with Clive Sellick and June Thoburn) *What Works in Foster Care and Adoption?* (Barnardo's, 2004); and he has co-authored four books on working with children traumatised through child abuse, and a fifth volume, on family placement, will be published next year by Jessica Kingsley Publishing. In 2001 BAAF published his report into private fostering, *A Very Private Practice*. He has also published a report on kinship care and two reports on residential care for older people run by the Catholic Church, the latest of which, *The Length of Days: How Can the Church Meet the Challenges of an Ageing Society?*, was published earlier this year. He is a columnist for *YoungMinds Magazine*. He is a trustee of the Social Care Institute or Excellence and of the Michael Sieff Foundation, having previously been a member of the boards of Rainer and the Centre for Policy on Ageing. He was formerly editor of *Community Care* and has won several awards for journalism.

Acknowledgements

This book could never have been written without the women who allowed me to interview them. They must, of necessity, remain anonymous. I knew even when I contacted them that allowing me to talk to them would not be easy, given the strain and distress of what had happened to them and their families. Having spoken to them, I know now just how grateful I must be to them. They demonstrate that behind superficial appearances and assumption, as W.H. Auden wrote,

> There is always another story, there is more than meets
> The eye

I cannot, then, thank them too much for their willingness, honesty and reflection, which I hope they will agree shows in the outcome; and I hope that the main reason why they spoke to me – that others should understand – will be achieved.

I have also to thank the two men – "Graham Byers" and "Paul Carpenter" – who also allowed themselves to be interviewed. For reasons different from those of the women, agreement to undertake this was not easy for them, and again, having met them I must underline my gratitude, especially for their honesty and openness.

I would also like to thank the five women (who also must remain anonymous) who allowed me to attend one of the meetings of their Partners for Protection group. This placed some flesh on, and provided understanding of, what I had read and been told about how the group's work. Something of that day is reflected in Chapter 4 about Mosaic, which is a project run by Barnardo's.

My gratitude cannot be repaid to Carol Butler, service manager Shelagh Scott, senior practitioner, and Richard Jackson, senior practitioner, all at Mosaic. Their conversations were invaluable in helping me to understand their work and the situations of those to whom I spoke and the many who stood behind them whom I did not meet but who have been helped over the years by the project. Carol, Shelagh and Richard also helped me with many questions during the writing of the book and Carol read and commented on Chapters 2 and 4.

Also at Mosaic, Tricia Carney, service administrator, helped with administrative tasks (not the least of which was making contact with women whom I might interview, even though they sometimes proved difficult to trace). Valerie Goodwill, service secretary, who, in so accurately transcribing the recordings, did one of the most important and difficult jobs and allowed me more fully to concentrate on interviewing and writing.

Invaluable in this, too, was Chris Hanvey, director of operations UK, Barnardo's, who had the idea three years ago that Mosaic's work might lend itself to a book. I refined this into the idea of a book about the female partners of child sex offenders, which would make use of Mosaic's work. Chris has offered his interest and support during the research and writing.

However, this might have remained just an interesting prospect had not a family trust provided the necessary funding to allow me to turn it into a book. Thanks must be given to Clare Parsons, who was then advising the trust, for being so enthusiastic from my first mention of the idea. (Our chance meeting, which took place before the book had ever been thought of, proves that serendipity can produce more results than an armful of funding applications.)

I have also to thank Barnardo's for meeting my travel and accommodation costs.

Great thanks are due to the staff of the NSPCC Library in London who unfailingly answered every question and found every reference and, on occasion, gave me a desk to allow me to follow these up. Their help reveals again what a superb (and free) resource the NSPCC makes available to researchers and writers.

Linda Ward, Professor of Disability and Social Policy, Norah Fry Research Centre, University of Bristol, meticulously read the introduction and Chapters 1, 2, 3 and 4. Her keen eye and helpful comments (again) saved me from many a stylistic infelicity and helped me to avoid intellectual pitfalls.

I must especially acknowledge Roger Kennington, Senior Probation Officer and Project Coordinator of the Sexual Behaviour Unit, National Probation Service Northumbria. He was not only kind enough to read Chapter 3 but, in so doing, he explained in great detail points where I was guilty of misinterpretation. He thereby made a substantial contribution to the final draft of that chapter. Roger also assisted with several useful references.

Jacquelyn Burke, Safeguarding Manager at Barnardo's, kindly read Chapter 1 and made helpful suggestions, as did Donald Findlater, Director of Research and Development of the Lucy Faithfull Foundation, with regard to Chapters 1 and 3. His colleague, Carol Geere, the foundation's media and communications manager, made those chapters available to colleagues and garnered their comments.

Last, but certainly not least, my thanks to Grace McInnes, my editor at Routledge, who encouraged me by taking to the idea immediately, even when I had not raised the funds to undertake the work, and who has offered advice along the way.

This book would be very much the less without such varied help and encouragement, but it goes without saying that I alone am responsible for opinion and any errors of fact and interpretation.

A note on terminology

Although this book is about men who have abused children, and most child sexual abuse is perpetrated by men against girls, women also abuse children[1] and boys are abused. Because of this and for ease of reading I have chosen to refer to the victims of sexual abuse as "she" and perpetrators as "he" unless referring to specific cases and individuals.

I have also avoided using the term "paedophile" because it is far too loosely used, even by professionals, as a synonym for child sex offender and so contributes to the idea that men who sexually abuse children are a homogenous group. (Indeed, one author, whom I will not name, is guilty of doing this throughout an otherwise helpful book.)[2]

I have used the words "offenders" and "sex offenders" as synonyms for "child sex offenders". When I have wanted to refer to other kinds of offender or offenders generally I have made this specific.

Introduction

There are three main parties in cases of child sexual abuse: the female partner of the offender, the offender and the child.[1] There is a deep inequality in how these parties are regarded and treated. It is common for the public to see child sexual abuse in stark shades of black and white, and this is appropriate in that the abuse of a child is always wrong. Most attention is given to child victims, because their situation is the most dreadful and severe. Much attention is also (rightly) focused on offenders.

The intention of this book, however, is to look at how child sex abuse affects the woman who is the partner of the perpetrator and whose child is often his victim. It is she who is the most neglected of the three parties. This neglect is reflected by the amount of literature devoted to each. The literature on child abuse – theory, practice, research – tends to be overwhelmingly about children as victims, understandably and rightly so. Many volumes, too, have been written about perpetrators. By contrast, there is very little about non-abusing mothers and female partners of sex offenders.

This neglect is also reflected in the most important area of concern: treatment. It is true that most children who have been abused do not receive adequate (if any) treatment and so may never fully recover from their experience, with often devastating consequences in later life. While most offenders never get to court, of those who do only a minority of offenders receive any kind of treatment and so they frequently return to the world with the experience of prison and not much more. The consequences of this can be devastating, by leading to further unsatisfactory and often abusive relationships and reoffending. But for both *some* victims and *some* perpetrators there is *some* treatment and, importantly, there is a widespread recognition that there is not enough treatment and that more ought to be made more widely available.

With mothers this is not the case. Even when innocent of any wrongdoing, they often not only suffer guilt by association with the offender, but are sometimes thought to be involved in the abuse, if only because "she must have known". Yet their needs are frequently dismissed or overlooked and no thought is given to addressing them. After all, what needs do they have? It is the child who has the greatest need and, after that, it is the offender who needs treatment, even within the confines of prison walls.

Yet these mothers are not only secondary victims, but also have a critical role to play in the protection of their children as well as in the child's recovery.

Offenders' partners are, then, frequently invisible, not only to the public but also to the agencies whose job it is to deal with abuse – the police, social workers, therapists and health service staff. So far as it is possible to tell, there only a few organisations specifically devoted to working with women in families affected by sexual abuse. It may be that there are even fewer actually working with the female partners of men who have sexually abused children.

The Lucy Faithful Foundation is possibly unique in working throughout the UK with the female partners of sex offenders. It also runs the Inform course specifically with partners and families of men who have accessed child pornography on the internet. This is an educational programme which provides advice and support to those affected by this crime. It offers ways to understand the crime and ways to keep children safe in the future.

In the late 1990s, the Foundation produced, at the request of the National Probation Service, an intervention programme for partners of men involved in the Thames Valley Sex Offender Treatment programme. While this sex offender treatment programme remains available for sex offenders across a third of England and Wales, the groupwork programme for partners is much less used – the victim of targets operating within the probation service. In autumn 2008 the foundation was due to implement an abbreviated programme, in collaboration with the Children's Services Department, Birmingham City Council, which will be evaluated by the University of Birmingham (Findlater 2008).

The Partners for Protection programme, in Newcastle-upon-Tyne, is run jointly by Barnardo's Mosaic project and the Sexual Behaviour Unit, created by Newcastle, North Tyneside and Northumberland NHS Mental Health Trust. The course runs for six hours a day, one day a week for eight weeks. It assesses the capacity of women whose partners have offended to protect their children and helps them to better protect them. (See Chapter 4 for a description of the programme.)

While the main purpose of this book is to allow women to tell their own stories in their own words, it was necessary to write four contextual chapters: on child sexual abuse; on offenders; a general analysis of what we know about the female partners of sex offenders; and a description of how the Partners for Protection programme works. Interviews with two offenders (one of them a partner) have also been included, to offer insights into their own experience and the nature of some offenders.

However, as has been said, the primary aim of this book is explain the situation of a woman whose partner commits a sexual offence against a child. Very commonly but not exclusively this may be the woman's own child. That child may be the offender's child also. Such abuse throws a spotlight on the dynamics of family relationships which have gone horribly wrong. What women feel in such circumstances, how they react, what happens to their relationships with partner, their child, other children, and other members of the family, the reactions of agencies like social work services and the police, as well as those of neighbours – all of these shape the new pattern of a woman's life, thoughts and feelings.

Each woman experiences what happens differently, and the reactions of all the women to whom I spoke are tempered by their experience of having attended the Partners for Protection programme. For all of them it was a welcome experience, even if some of them did not think it would be. Some refer to how it changed them for the better – they became more self-assured, more self-confident, better able to protect their children, more aware (or, in some cases, for the first time aware) of the stratagems of offenders, against which they now felt able better to be on their guard. Most offenders never appear before the courts (as is the case in the majority of the cases described here) and it is this that most seems to anger and frustrate the women. that justice is, literally, not done, that the man has "got away with it", that he has never paid the price. For most, even for those who seem to look most calmly at their experiences, this is what most prevents the ghost of what has happened being laid to rest.

My main aim, in writing this book has been to allow the women to have the opportunity to speak for themselves, so that their biographies, histories and experiences should be told unvarnished by an interviewer, unmediated by interpretation by the third party of the author. It is important to allow them to say in their own words what happened and how they and those closest to them have reacted to this, but this is necessary also for strong symbolic and actual reasons: because the voices of such women are seldom if ever heard.

I interviewed seven women between September 2007 and March 2008, each for about one and a half to two hours, at the offices of Mosaic. The interviews were fairly free flowing. Each of interviewees had been sent beforehand a list of topics which I hoped to discuss when we met, but I let them know that, of course, it was for them to tell me as much or as little as they chose. The two offenders were interviewed in March 2008, again at the Mosaic offices and for the same lenght of time. I went through the same procedures with them.

The recordings were transcribed and then edited by me to excise repetition and to give the stories the shape and sense of narrative that conversation does not always allow. However, this editing was subtle and not extensive because my guiding principle was that the stories belonged to the interviewees and they should tell them in their own way, as I have said. Questions and interventions were (mostly) omitted to add to the immediacy of what was being said. The transcripts were then sent to each interviewee, who could comment, add and subtract from the script as she chose. The changes were few and minor and what is presented here is what emerged from that process.

For obvious reasons, pseudonyms are used not only for the women and the men but for children, partners, former partners, friends and relatives, and any identifying details have been changed. These changes were agreed with the subjects.

The average age of the mothers to whom I spoke was 37 (ranging from 22 to 50) at the time of the interviews (ages given for all characters in the stories are also as they were at the time of the interview). All the women were white British, and six could be characterised as working class, using both their own occupations and those of their fathers as a guide. Four of them were in full- or part-time employment, while three were in receipt of benefits (one due to physical disability). Two were or had been married to the offender and five were or had been living with him. (I took a cohabiting man to be, effectively, a stepfather and his birth relatives to be, effectively, step uncles and so on.) At the time of interview two women hoped to reunite with their partners.

The mothers had an average of 2.5 children each (14 in all). Five of the mothers had children who were also children of the offender. Two of those children had been abused by the father and the other by the mother's partner. (One man's offence had been to access child pornography from the web. The exact number of images is not known but is believed to have run into thousands. There was no evidence that he had physically abused his children or any other children.) In one of these cases, the abused daughter eventually lived with a man who abused another child not known to him. Three of the 14 children had at one time been in the care of the local authority as a result of what had happened and they were still in care at the time of the interview.

The number of children known to have been directly abused by offenders was 11 and it was possible that two of the men had each also abused two other children. Two of the offenders abused two children who were not related to them (although one of those men had also abused a child to whom he was related).

One offender (the one who had viewed pornography) had served 13 months of a 32-months sentence, another received 2 years' probation (and a 2-year suspended sentence for an offence disclosed 14 years after it had taken place), and a third had received supervision, as his offence was committed when he was 13 years of age. Another died while committing one of his crimes. The rest of the men had no proceedings taken against them.

I offered the mothers four reasons why they might have agreed to take part in the interviews. The reasons were: to allow them to put their experience to use in some way; that they felt the need to be believed, to be heard or to have their experienced recognised; to tell their story to someone; and to help others to understand. Three said that their reason was to help others understand, two others gave that same reason but also said that they wanted to use their experience in some way; and two agreed with all the reasons. (When I asked the men for their reasons for participating, both said that it was to counter media and popular stereotypes of sex offenders, a choice I had not offered them.)

In all of this work and more I was helped considerably by the existence of the Mosaic project. Not only was I able to draw on the experience and expertise of its staff who run the Partners for Protection programme for offenders' partners, but also I was able, through Mosaic's good offices, to make contact with the women and men who eventually agree to be interviewed.

It might be argued that those to whom I spoke (women and men) were not "typical", in that they were self-selecting and all the women had taken part in the Partners for Protection course (some at first reluctantly), while one of the men had participated in a programme for offenders. Also, for the majority of women in their situation there would have been no such help. However, the positive outcome of this was that the course had given them a greater insight into what had happened to themselves as mothers and people, which enhanced what they were able to relate.

Self-selecting and willing to be interviewed as the women may have been, the evidence from such research and writing as there has been about women whose partners sexually abuse children suggests that the subjects in this book are pretty typical. As with the many thousands like them, they have suffered family tragedy, shock, pain and disruption. They will have had to face self-doubt and self-recrimination. They will have had to cope with conflict and confusing emotions, and the reactions of family, friends, neighbours and others. They have had to think deeply about the actions of someone whom they may have trusted and loved and what those actions now mean to that relationship. And, finally, they will have had to cope with the needs of their children, who may have been abused or who, if not direct victims themselves, will have suffered the consequences of their father or their mother's partner having abused another child. In these aspects and others my seven female interviewees confirm the experiences of those who have been the subject of research and to whom I refer elsewhere, more generally, in the book.

The mothers to whom I spoke (including the five I met in their group) also openly acknowledged that they had learned from attending the Partners for Protection programme and were the better for acquiring that knowledge. However, the flow of information is not all one way. Society, too, requires education generally about child sexual abuse and, specifically, about women whose partners are sexual offenders: as is said elsewhere, it is the ignorance of the public which can often lead to mothers becoming secondary victims through social ostracism and having their homes attacked. Likewise, professionals need to know more about vulnerable women, because it is not only the child but her mother, too, who requires protection, support and guidance. To understand the emotions and mental processes of a woman in such a situation is not easy; they are not straightforward and even she is not always able to understand and manage them. The dynamic of conflicting feelings often described in these interviews is but one insight, gained from one project, into what professionals and society need to face and understand.

Understanding the wider context in which these stories are told is important, but what is also important in this book is what those mothers can tell the rest of us about what happened to them, their families and their children, and how they reflect on those experiences.

1 Children, sexual abuse and its effects

A cultural understanding of child sexual abuse

The death of Maria Colwell in East Sussex in 1973 at the hands of her step-father threw a glaring light on the physical abuse of children, which has yet to be dimmed (Department of Health and Social Security 1974). It gave renewed impetus to discussions, agitation, research, practice development, media coverage (sensationalist and otherwise), policy initiatives, and the restructuring of services which continues today. Long before some other professional groups became the subject of media and public scrutiny, social work was propelled into an arena to which it was not accustomed, a situation which still obtains all these years later.

Maria Colwell's death came three years after the creation of social services departments, which had seemed to signal a new dawn for social work. Nearly 30 years earlier, in 1945, the death of 13-year-old Denis O'Neill, beaten and starved by his foster father, had led to the Curtis report and the decision to create children's departments, that were later to be subsumed by those very the social services departments (Douglas and Philpot 1998). More than 50 years later the murder of Victoria Climbe by her great aunt and her aunt's lover in 2000 provoked the inquiry by Lord Laming which, in time, led indirectly to the abolition of the social services departments and the creation of local authority children's services departments separate from those for adults (Department of Health and the Home Office 2003).

Few children suffer only one form of abuse. The deaths of Denis O'Neill and Maria Colwell drew wide attention to physical abuse and neglect, as that of Victoria Climbe was to do. This was not wholly surprising in that the care of children had been so much shaped by those who had been determined to tackle these very social ills. The great children's charities, like Barnardo's (Rose 1987), NCH (Philpot 1994), the Church of England Central Home for Waifs and Strays Society (now the Children's Society) and the NSPCC, had been founded in the latter part of the 19th century to tackle the great evils of child neglect, physical abuse and abandonment.

In the last 20 years or so sexual abuse has come to the forefront in terms of professional concern and media and public interest. Indeed, it is arguable that this emphasis has now tended to overshadow issues of physical abuse and neglect. The definition of sexual abuse is something which changes from culture to culture, from period to period. Sanderson (2004) cites deMause (1976, 1991, 1992, 1993, 1998, 2002) as having found historical evidence of sexual abuse which has not been recognised as such because of the prevailing attitudes toward children at different times.

But we do not need to look at the past to understand how cultural norms affect how the treatment of children is viewed. In Chile and Mexico today, for example, the age of sexual consent is 12, which is two years below the age fixed by our Victorian ancestors in England. In other modern societies as diverse as Spain, North Korea and South Korea the age of consent is 13, while young people in Denmark, Sweden and France are able to consent to sexual intercourse when they become 15. In the United States the age of consent differs from state to state so that, for example, in New York it is 17 and in California it is 18. In Northern Ireland, a part of the UK, it is 17. Bolivia holds to 17, while Vietnam and Egypt have legislated for 18 and Tunisia for 20 years of age (*The Guardian* 2005).

Some sexual practices are acceptable in some places but abominated in others. Some African and Middle Eastern countries allow female genital circumcision, which is illegal in the USA and the UK, although there is evidence that operations still occur there. Sanderson (2004) quotes the World Health Organisation as estimating that between 130 and 140 million children in the world today have been subjected to this operation. In many countries marriage between children, and often marriage of a child to an adult, continues and in Egypt marriage between brothers and sisters is permitted. Elsewhere, temple maidens still exist: young girls provide sexual services to worshippers. The masturbation of boys to make them "manly" is accepted in some parts of India, while it is done to girls to make them "sleep well" (deMause 1976, 1991, 1993, 1998, 2002 quoted by Sanderson 2004). In some African countries, sex with a female child or young girl who is a virgin is believed to cure sexually transmitted diseases, an idea reaching back to ancient notions of the purity of children. In the age of AIDS/HIV this supposed antidote or preventative has taken on what is, literally, a deadly topicality. Again, older ideas of child sacrifice can be seen revived in the idea of ritual abuse, which has gained some attention in the UK, although there must remain some doubt as to how "genuine" such rituals are as opposed to being used to frighten children into submission.

Increasing attention, in Europe at least, is now being given to child prostitution with its often attendant evil of child trafficking. However, children do not have to be taken across borders or "trafficked" for them to be ensnared in the trade: it is believed that there are 300,000 child prostitutes in the United States and 200,000 in Thailand, the country with which it is most commonly associated. Sanderson (2004) claims that 14 per cent of Asian countries' GNP can be attributed to child prostitution through the sex tourism trade. In Britain there are thought to be 5,000 children in the sex trade and in France 8,000 (Sanderson 2004).

The sex trade can cross over with child pornography: children working as prostitutes will often be used in the making of pornographic movies. Internet and mobile phone technology has facilitated the spread and availability of pornography in a way which makes it now very difficult to detect and check effectively. By contrast, not many years ago pornography could only be obtained by visiting certain addresses or by having it sent from abroad or importing it oneself, which allowed its detection by customs officials. Pornographic images of children can now be had at the touch of a button in the privacy of one's own home.

The definition of abuse through pornography has been slower to develop than the technology which makes it so readily and easily available. It has been said (and not only self-servingly by those who make use of it) that viewing pornography in this way is "safe" and "victim free", but it is obvious that anyone making use of these sites is colluding in the abuse perpetrated against the children who are being shown. Buying, selling or otherwise disseminating and obtaining pornographic videos, photographs, DVDs and films in which children, sometimes no more than babies, feature are no less actual forms of abusive activities than other forms of abuse. These are real children and this is not acting. These are not victimless crimes, and sentencing policies in the UK have now begun to reflect that fact, as has the public disapproval of those who take part in such activities.

What is child sexual abuse?

As we can see, there are inconsistencies in definitions of sexual abuse associated with social and cultural constructions. However, while the age of consent differs in many, often seemingly similar societies, key criteria concerning the imbalance of power between victim and perpetrator, lack of consent and the inability to give consent must remain central. This book follows the definitions current in the UK:

> Definitions of child sexual abuse should acknowledge the abuse of power and trust; that it is carried out by an adult for his [sic] own sexual gratification; and that children cannot give free and informed consent to sexual acts with adults.
>
> (Reid 1989: 1)

The widely used definition by Kempe and Kempe meets Reid's definitional purposes:

> Sexual abuse is defined as the involvement of dependent, developmentally immature children and adolescents in sexual activities that they do not fully comprehend, to which they are unable to give informed consent, or that violate the social taboos of family roles.
>
> (Kempe and Kempe 1978: 60)

A quarter of a century after this definition was formulated the Department of Health and the Home Office offered another, which focuses on the nature of activities undertaken:

Forcing or enticing a child or young person to take part in sexual activities whether or not the child is aware of what is happening. The activities may involve physical contact, including penetrative (eg, rape or buggery) and non-penetrative acts. They may include non-contact activities such as involving children in looking at, or in the production of pornographic material, or watching sexual activities, or encouraging children to behave in sexually inappropriate ways.

(Department of Health and Home Office 2003)

While babies can be abused as can 15-year-olds, the age group most at risk is those aged 5 to 12 years (Sanderson 2004). Sanderson also has a list of 18 "non-contact behaviours" and 20 "contact behaviours" involved in sexual abuse and adds others like grooming, voyeurism, fondling and exhibitionism. Perpetrators may include family members, professionals whom children are likely to have contact with (for example, teachers and youth club workers) and others who have contact with children (for example, baby sitters), as well as people who may know the child, like shopkeepers (Sanderson 2004: 46).

All this serves to demonstrate that what we call sexual abuse can take many forms, happen in many places and include a wide range of activities, and that offenders are extraordinarily varied.

In middle-class families child sexual abuse can be often covered up, not talked about, and hidden in different ways. Indeed, the "respectability" of such homes can instil the belief that such things "do not happen" in such families. These families, too, are far less likely to be known to the authorities – like the police and social workers – and so there is less opportunity for such outsiders to suspect that something may be afoot. But, there is no evidence that sexual abuse is confined to any one social class: it occurs within a wider context of family dysfunction. However, abuse is more likely to occur in families where there is privation and deprivation, and much takes place in families that are chaotic. This is where children experience a frequently revolving pageant of adults who come into and go from their lives: when a parent changes partners, new sets of relatives, formal or informal, appear. A partner who lives in or who enters the family home may themselves have other children who are then step- or half-brothers and sisters. Such complexity would be bewildering to an adult, let alone a child who is not only emotionally underdeveloped but is also not the agent of such change. What is happening to her is being caused by others. Indeed, she may have only the haziest understanding of who these others are, even if they are formally related.[1]

The extent of abuse

It is difficult to arrive at firm figures about how extensive sexual abuse is because, like rape, much of it goes unreported or is only reported many years later, when the victims are adults and when the possibility of conviction (never high) is considerably less likely. Cawson *et al.* (2000), in perhaps the most exhaustive, reliable and widely accepted study, found that 1 per cent of children aged under 16 had experienced sexual abuse by a parent or carer and another 3 per cent by another relative during childhood. To this must be added the 5 per cent said to be abused as children by an adult stranger or someone whom they have just met.[2] However, the most common perpetrators of oral or penetrative sexual abuse within the family are brothers or stepbrothers (38 per cent), fathers (28 per cent), uncles (14 per cent), stepfathers (13 per cent), cousins (8 per cent), grandfathers (6 per cent) and mothers (4 per cent) (Cawson *et al.* 2000).

A much smaller scale study by Hooper (1992) of mothers whose children had been abused offers an insight into who are perpetrators. Her 15 mothers all had children who had been sexually abused by members of the household or "non-resident kin" (not all of whom were adults). The abusers were a son (1); husband (4); ex-husband (3); ex-cohabitee (2); relative of ex-cohabitee (2); mother's father (1); and ex-husband and stepfather to child (2).

According to ChildLine (2003) both boys and girls are sexually abused but girls are more commonly abused by a ratio of nearly 1:4.[3] Cawson *et al.*'s (2000) gender breakdown suggests that 11 per cent of boys under 16 and 21 per cent of girls aged under 16 have been sexually abused. Another study (Grubin 1998) found that 60–70 per cent of sex offenders against children targeted only girls, 20–33 per cent only boys, and about 10 per cent targeted either sex. According to Grubin, "about 80 per cent of offences take place in the home of either the offender or the victim".

Available figures on convictions for sexual abuse against children are further complicated by the high percentage of perpetrators who are other children and young (mainly adolescent) people. Lovell (2002) says that there is "a broad consensus" that they make up between 25 to 35 per cent of perpetrators.

Between 1985 and 2001, recorded offences of gross indecency with children more than doubled but the percentage of convictions fell from 42 per cent to 19 per cent. Stuart and Baines (2004) suggest that fewer than 1 in 50 sex offenders receive a criminal conviction. Although some of these unconvicted and unreported offences will have been committed by perpetrators who have been convicted for other offences, that still means that a very large majority of offences against children are not reported. If they are reported, the perpetrator may never get to court. If he does, there is a good chance that he will escape conviction.

Public discussion about child sex abuse is made more difficult because of traditional fear of strangers. It distorts public understanding of who actually abuses children. This may be accounted for, to a degree, by cultural notions of the safe family against the threatening outside world and the kind of external threats exemplified in fairy stories like "Little Red Riding Hood". Even if such fears are vestigial, they are exacerbated by popular media headlines about the "paedo", "sex abuse monster", "pervert", and such like which tend to high-light strangers who have committed acts against children. It is not difficult to understand the viewpoint of some journalists: stories of children who are abducted by severely disturbed and sometimes repeat offenders and are found to be the victims of sexual murder make more interesting "copy" than the horrors which the majority of child sex abuse victims suffer within the four walls of their own homes at the hands of their parents, other relatives and family friends. Media coverage of sexual offences against children can, therefore, grossly mislead and militate against proper public understanding of the issue.

The truth is prosaic: the facts show indisputably that a child is in much more danger in her own home, in the "care" of those whom she knows, than she ever is from a stranger in the street. The abuse could be carried out by a family member or family friend, and this includes, of course, children and young people who abuse other children.

Abuse is also often systematic and continuing. It may last for months or even years. Some children are abused into young adulthood and the abuse only ends when they leave the family home, although even that is sometimes not the case.

How children react to sexual abuse

Each child will react differently to sexual abuse and the most we can say, in general terms, is that its effect will very often (but not always) be profoundly damaging. How damaging and in what ways will depend on many things: the age at which abuse took place; the extent and nature of the abuse; how long it lasted; how isolated the child was within her family (for example, whether other children were abused and whether this was known to her); who the abuser was and her relationship with him; the prevailing family dynamic (that is, the relationship of the abuser, who may or may not have been the child's father, and his partner, and the relationship of the child and her mother); and, importantly, how her disclosing what happened was dealt with and the help which she received. Whatever the effects, it is probably true, as one victim said, that "it creeps into every part of your life" (quoted in Mudaly and Goddard 2006).

Whom *do* children tell? Many children never tell anyone, and this is the case even when they grow to adulthood. One in four children is thought to disclose what happened to them at the time when it occurred, and another quarter later, but just under a third (31 per cent) never tell. Of those who do disclose, more than half (55 per cent) tell a friend, 29 per cent their mother or stepmother, and 11 per cent their father. Brothers and sisters are told by 13 per cent, and social workers by 2 per cent. Seven per cent let the police know, 5 per cent inform a teacher and 1 per cent phone a helpline (Featherstone and Evans 2004).

The NSPCC's National Commission of Inquiry into the Prevention of Child Abuse, which advertised for people to testify, found from the 1,121 responses it received that 32 per cent had told someone and 31 per cent of these had told an adult. For 13 per cent of those who had contacted the inquiry or an agony aunt (the inquiry used "agony aunt" columns as one way of reaching people), it was the first time that they had disclosed what had happened to them (Wattam and Woodward 1996).

An analysis of the 32 per cent who told the inquiry that they had told someone, revealed that 34 per cent told their mothers when they were children but 13 per cent did not do so until they were adults. Sixteen per cent told a friend or boyfriend when a child; 5 per cent did so in adulthood. Twenty-four per cent told partners and spouses, while 10 per cent told other relatives when they were children, and 8 per cent did so when they were adults. Three per cent told counsellors when they were children and 15 per cent did so when they were adults. Two per cent told a doctor when they were children and 6 per cent did so when they were adults. Seven per cent told the police in childhood and 4 per cent when adults. Seven per cent told teachers, while 5 per cent were children when they told social workers and 1 per cent were adults. Two per cent told their fathers when they were children; none did when they were grown up. Of the 2 per cent who told "others", all did so as adults. It was not clear to whom 10 per cent had disclosed as children, and 20 per cent as adults (Wattam and Woodward 1996).

Female friends of the victim and her sisters were more likely to be told of assaults than were mothers. (Agencies learned of even fewer cases than did mothers.) However, it was more likely that a mother would be told when a girl was abused by an adult. When the abuser was under the age of 18, females of the same age as the victim were more likely to know (Kelly *et al.* 1991).

Sexual abuse presents a child with desperate dilemmas which place her in a terrible double bind when it comes to disclosure. When she tells what has happened to her, the abuse will end but its effects remain. But disclosure itself will have consequences. For example, how will a child defend herself from the wounding accusations which she may face from those affected by her allegation? She will naturally feel responsible for some results which may flow from her actions: the offender, whom she may love, may go to prison. What she has revealed may cause a rift in the family; a prison sentence may split it asunder. It is not only the perpetrator, his partner (usually her mother) and the child who are affected, but also other family members: any brothers and sisters, grandparents, uncles and aunts and cousins. Some may think she did right to disclose, some may not believe her, some may think she is exaggerating and ask why did she not leave well alone.

Disclosure may provoke a variety of feelings in the child's mother (as we shall see later), which may include a sense of loss (for partner and united family), guilt (at her own failure to spot what was occurring), and anger (at herself, her partner, even her child). Being placed in care may be the outcome of the allegations for the child and some or all of her brothers and sisters.

Doubt and self-doubt may also affect children as the drama unfolds. As Pughe and Philpot explain:

> it is highly likely that at some point the child will again suffer great panic and fear. She may even question the wisdom of what she has done and has caused to happen. Was I to blame? What did *I* do to make dad want to act sexually with me? Everything may come to seem out of control; she may wish she could go back in time and leave things as they were, coming to believe that bad as they were, they are not as bad as what is happening now.

Self-doubt or mounting confusion are now the child's companions and it is likely that she will condemn herself and question whether the abuse really warranted all the fuss and interference – was it *really* that bad? – or could ever justify the dreadful drama of the courtroom and the consequences which flow from it. She may well weigh in her mind whether her need to put a stop to the abuse is worth the consequences: the family riven, she and her brothers and sisters in care, her father in prison, her mother alone.

(Pughe and Philpot 2007: 16–17)

A child is not healed or made better if she has to go through the criminal justice system and to court. She may have to appear and give evidence of the most traumatic kind against her parent, but sometimes she will have waited as long as 18 months before being called upon to do so. Plotnikoff and Wolfson (2005) interviewed 50 child witnesses, aged from 7 to 17 years, 32 of whom appeared in sex offence cases. Not surprisingly, they often felt intimidated in court. Some said that appearing as a witness could be as traumatic as the original abuse. Just under half said that they had been accused of lying and more than half said that they had been very upset, distressed or angry. A fifth of those said that they had cried, felt sick or sweated.

Even the outcome of a successful conviction may leave the child feeling "the sinking mud of despair" (Hunter 2001: 79).

The conflicts, dilemmas and confusion which can beset a child in such a situation are not easily resolved and neither will they necessarily be static. What she feels may change from one moment to the next. What feels right at one time may not feel so the next. Perhaps the most complicated emotions will be those exhibited toward the perpetrator. He may be someone whom she loved and now both loves and hates. She may not want him to be taken from the family home. What she wants is the abuse to stop. Again, Pughe and Philpot explain:

All of this makes the child see nothing but a precipice and below it a dark, unfathomable valley. To escape this, she may see the answer as the wish, the deep, deep desire to give in to the urge to go into emotional free-flow. She may crave to feel nothing at all, to become numb or able to switch off all the noise and for her world to fall silent. She may experience thoughts and sensations that appear to make her feel she is about to break into small pieces. She may feel the threat of annihilation, an almost literal sense of that "going to pieces" that so many of us express as a feeling when things seem beyond our control. She lacks anchor, direction, and any sense of grounding or rootedness. This wish to let go, to become as nothing, then, seems a way out.

(Pughe and Philpot 2007: 17)

Children who are taken into care as a consequence of their disclosure suffer an additional discontinuity in their lives, another rupture of the familiar, which can have severe negative consequences for them and for their behaviour. But negative behaviour does not result only when an abused child goes into care. Any abused child's perceptions of herself, her world and others will become distorted. Confusion may reign, a sense of self-worth plummet. As a result, the child may become aggressive, detached and withdrawn, and unpredictable in her behaviour. Temper tantrums, kicking, spitting and biting are other ways in which she may manifest her complicated emotions, as are self-harm and self-destructiveness to the point of being suicidal. These children may abscond, trash the place where they are living – the foster carer's home, the children's home – or steal. They may destroy what is important to them. Their psychosexual development has been grossly distorted, so that their behaviour toward staff, foster carers, other children and even complete strangers can be highly eroticised (Rymaszewska and Philpot 2006: 34).

The consequences of abuse bear brutally on emotions of people too young to comprehend them. The act of abuse brings with it physical pain and deep emotional distress. But it also dramatically affects a child's personality and understanding of herself and her world: she will have a sense of loss and feel rejected. She may be lonely. She will experience doubts about others and herself. She loses trust in others, even those who are now there to help her. Dislocation and rootlessness may result for some of these children and entry into the care system may only serve to increase this.

Sexual abuse, then, raises all manner of conflicting emotions in children, many of whom will not understand what has been done to them or why. Mixed with this will be feelings of guilt and self-reproach, and how they feel – negatively and positively – about the perpetrator. It is no surprise, then, Cawson *et al.* (2000) found, that in fact three-quarters (72 per cent) of sexually abused children did not tell anyone about the abuse at the time. Just over a quarter (27 per cent) told someone later, while about a third (31 per cent) still had not told anyone about their experiences by early adulthood.

Sadly, too few children receive the specialised and highly professional care needed to recover from the trauma they will have experienced. As Moore (1992) has said: "Disclosure without therapy is the second rape of the child." Life after the care system, for those who enter it, can be one of drift, difficulty in settling, and unstable and promiscuous relationships which may involve abuse, and crime. But there are abused children who are assisted by the care system and there are many others who do not enter it because they remain within their families – with their mother. It is the experience and role of the mother, the partner of the offender, which is the focus of this book and it is to her experiences to which we now turn.

2　A mother's lot

Chris Roberts takes a carefully preserved newspaper cutting from an envelope, unfolds it and shows it to me with a certain satisfaction. It is the story of the trial and sentencing of her former partner, Sean Francis. Even though no charges were brought against him for the sexual abuse of their then 3-year-old daughter, Chantelle, Chris gains some satisfaction that he is serving two years for threatening behaviour in a very different kind of case.

When her partner was arrested by police for questioning about his alleged sexual abuse of their child, Chris was taken to a women's refuge, while her daughter went into temporary foster care. Returning to collect clothes, Chris found their house had been ransacked by neighbours and that what they could not destroy had been stolen. The ceilings had been deliberately damaged so that rain had flooded in. The neighbours said that they wanted to wreak their revenge on Francis. Chris finishes talking about him by saying: "I just cannot wait till he's six feet under. I would go to his funeral just to make sure he was buried and that would be the only reason."

Rachel Bond's husband, Tom, served 16 months of his 32-month sentence for accessing hundreds of horrifying images of children on the internet, including images of torture and sexual violence. A few days after her husband was charged, Rachel went, as usual, to her church in the small town in which she lives. At the end of the service, she asked everyone to stay behind as she had an announcement to make. She told her fellow parishioners what had happened. Now, her husband has since been released from prison and she has welcomed him back into their home to remake their lives with their two children. She says:

> I wanted us to be a family again but I think that I had it in my head from quite early on. I don't think you know how you're going to feel about things until it's upon you really.
>
> It's just, what do you believe about this person? Do you believe they have done this awful thing? Absolutely, yes!
>
> I could have walked away, I could still walk away. Do I think that's the right thing to do and do I think that's the right thing to do for me? I don't think that's the right thing to do for him. This is not in order of priority but do I think it's not the right thing for Mark and Sarah [their children]?

I don't think it's the right thing for Matthew and Beth [her adult step-children]. I don't think it's the right thing for his dad. But if I didn't feel as confident about the past, if I had any kind of unanswered questions, then I don't think I would feel like this. If Tom had laid hands on Matthew, Beth, Mark or Sarah I wouldn't feel like this and I wouldn't be making this decision and if there were ever any repeat or any suggestion of repetition of any of this sort of behaviour then I wouldn't be sticking around.

These are two women who have lived two very different lives with two very different men, the fathers of their children. Yet such differences – or the kind of sexual abuse in which the men were involved – do not wholly account for their differing reactions. Indeed, as she says, Rachel believed that she might not have been so determined to remake her family life with her husband had he abused their children, appalling though she finds his crime. But the extreme difference in their reactions illustrates the spectrum of responses of women whose partners have been involved in the sexual abuse of children.

Discovery and reaction

Sex offenders do not necessarily offend against their own children. However, when this does happen, it may suggest a single point in time when a child tells all, when all becomes suddenly clear. In fact, matters are rarely so straightforward. And neither is it straightforward when a woman discovers that her partner has offended against someone else's child.

Being told what has happened is not the same as understanding, or even accepting it. Sexual abuse is something that happens between people; its discovery is not analogous to other kinds of discovery. Added to this is the issue of believing – if a mother is told what has happened can she (in the first instance at least) believe it? Is it possible to think that her partner would do this to their child or to another child? Could this person, whom she believes she knows so well (and loves), really look at such dreadful images on a computer screen for some kind of enjoyment? The immediate anger of some women is to be contrasted with the (not unnatural) belief of others not so much that the child is lying – though some women will believe that to be so – but that there must be some mistake, some misunderstanding. To either of these reactions may be added the woman's own feelings about her relationship with her partner.

Those untouched by sexual abuse (even professionals) may expect a mother's response to be different from that which she exhibits. As Ovaris (1991) puts it:

What would be the expected response of a mother to such an encounter? An enthusiastic or calm acceptance of the information as true? A spontaneous affirmation that her husband could be molesting his own child? Immediate validation of her daughter's *alleged* statements about her father? The answer to all of these questions is "no". (p. 11)

Whether conscious or otherwise, one immediate response is of dilemma which touches deeply upon a woman's emotional and moral responses. She is being asked, in effect, to choose: not to believe her child, whom she loves, and support her, and to continue to believe a man whom she loves. How she reacts to this will be, in some respects, influenced by the kind of relationship she has had with her partner. Within that relationship are the questions about the part he has played in her life (what power, for example, did he exercise?); the nature of their intimacy; and how much trust they shared.

How women react in the short term will depend partly on the way in which the news came to them. Rachel Bond had a knock on the door from the police on a bright, sunny day when she was playing in the garden with one of her small children. Ann Baker (who is also interviewed in this book) had a night out with two of her daughters which ended with her hearing that her husband had died while sexually abusing a friend of the third daughter in their home – and then, on the day of her father's funeral, that daughter revealed that she, too, had been abused by her father for years. For Clare Truman (another interviewee), it was the day when a police officer and a social worker turned up at the home she shared with her partner to reveal three allegations against him of sexually abusing children, one of them his (but not her) son.

Reactions, too, will depend on the relationship with the offender – how stable the relationship; what suspicions (if any) the mother may have had; whether there was any suggestion (or evidence) in the past of similar offences. But horror, disbelief, anger, pain and panic – even when the news is confirmation of the vaguest of suspicions – are common. A sense of security and trust in the other person may be shattered by the news, and even when the offence is not against children in the family, the family is violated. Even women who are utterly shocked that the man they thought they knew so well could do something like this still question themselves. Was there something, some revealing behaviour, which they missed? Was there something lacking in her that made him do it? Was it her fault in some way? Surely she would have seen something? All these are common reactions.

A woman who has enjoyed a loving and stable relationship with her partner may be all the more shocked at the news of the allegation of abuse because, it may be argued, the disclosure has come as a shock, a bolt from the blue, something never expected. She may doubt the truth of the allegation or think that there has been a misunderstanding. However, a woman who has been in a relationship with a man who has been, say, abusive to her, and about whom she has had her suspicions, might be expected to react immediately in support of her child when she is told of the abuse, because this is something that she might have expected, something that might have lingered, as a suspicion or fear, in the recesses of her psyche. However, her "clear cut" response will be hampered by her own guilt: why did she ever enter the relationship and why did she not end it?

These are some reasons why professionals cannot expect, as Ovaris (1991) says, that a mother "will immediately respond as a competent and co-operative 'colleague', focusing all her energy and attention on the well-being of her child".

Hooper and Humphreys (1998) discovered that women's support for their children can be categorised as neither supportive nor unsupportive but tends to fluctuate in tune with their own emotional distress and the way in which discovery has disrupted their lives. And a supportive mother may not receive an unconditional, positive response from her child in return: she may be greeted by anger, guilt, blame and a sense of betrayal.

Discovery can come in different ways. A woman may suspect her partner, challenge him, and he then confesses. Her child may tell her and she may confront him, with the same result. She may suspect, and ask the child who then tells all. She may come across letters or a diary. She may discover the partner abusing the child by coming home at the "wrong" time or being awake when he believed she was asleep. The police and social workers may turn up at the front door. (For a more detailed picture of how children disclose and to whom, see Chapter 1 and below).

Plummer (2006) surveyed 125 non-abusive mothers of sexually abused children who were primarily Caucasian and African-Americans living in a Midwestern state of the United States. She found that mothers first came to learn by being told (42 per cent) or as a result of their child's behaviour (15 per cent). Half of the women had a sense that "something was not quite right" before they knew about the abuse. Sixty-six per cent sought clarification about what was happening by talking to their child or by watching things more closely (39 per cent). The evidence that they found most convincing was what the child said (74 per cent), her behaviour (66 per cent) and the child's emotional reactions (60 per cent). Twenty-one per cent of mothers became increasingly uncertain when the abuser denied what had happened.

Humphreys (1992) described mothers whose children disclose as being within a "continuum of belief". They acted as if they believed but "vacillated between degrees of cognitive belief and emotional acceptance of the reality of abuse" (Clothier 2008). When Myer (1985) looked at a group of women whose children disclosed abuse, half of them responded protectively; a quarter were immobilised, although not disbelieving; and a quarter rejected their children. Myer's explanation for denial is that it is part of the classic reaction to grief, formulated by Kubler-Ross (1970), in reaction to those facing death. This is a dynamic process of stages, beginning with denial and isolation, followed by anger; bargaining; depression; and, at last, acceptance.[1] Hooper and Humphreys (1998) report that women "frequently" spoke of being isolated when attempting to support their child.

According to Massat and Lundy (1998), the costs or losses which a woman experiences may, in some cases, influence how supportive she is after disclosure. The authors posited the kinds of potential loss suffered by mothers as being those of the loss of the partner; disruptions to family and friends; loss of income; a change of home (this happened to half of those to whom the authors spoke); and "vocational", which may be taken to refer to having to change jobs or to seek work if the partner had been the breadwinner.

At this time, too, mothers will experience a spread of emotions toward their child which range from anger to sympathy. However, negative reactions appear to be rare: Gomes-Schwarz *et al.* (1990) reported that 90 per cent of mothers displayed moderate to strong concern for their children. We know that if children experience a mother's support after abuse they will demonstrate an increase in positive perceptions of themselves and a decrease in the symptoms of depression (Morrison and Clavenna-Valleroy 1998).

In a maelstrom of emotions and complications, there are further complications when the offending partner is not the child's biological father. Reactions here will be determined, in part, by the quality of the relationship between the separated couple. Blame and guilt may flow back freely from one to the other and their personal differences be given vent through what has happened. This may be further complicated if a biological father is on hand to seek a change in the child's living arrangements and wants her to live with him.

Mothers' longer-term responses

Women's responses to both the abuser and the child are very likely to say something about their previous relationships with each. For example, Hooper (1992: 5) quotes several studies to show that women are "somewhat less likely" to be supportive when the abuser is their current partner than when he is in any other relationship to them (what other relationship is not specified). Everson *et al.* (1989) suggest that mothers whose partners confirm the abuse are more likely to be consistently supportive of their abused children; when the partner denies his wrongdoing, the mother is less likely to believe what her child has said. But a partner who denies abuse can place a woman in the situation of seeming to choose between her child and her partner. Everson *et al.* (1989) say that there is an inverse relationship between a mother's support for her child and how recent is her relationship with the perpetrator. If she is no longer married to, or living with him, the mother is likely to be significantly more supportive to the child.

Women who have had a caring relationship with their children are most likely to be concerned and protective; those who have felt hostile or overburdened are more likely to be angry and unsupportive. Thus, just as mothers can aid recovery, so they can impede it, although it is only a minority of mothers who are not supportive to their child (Hooper 1992).

Research from the United States (Sirles and Franke 1989) indicates that several factors contribute to how a woman reacts to reported abuse. These are the age of the victim; the nature of the abuse; the presence of the mother in the home when the abuse took place; the relationship of victim to offender; prior abuse of the child; and alcohol abuse by the perpetrator. But the writers add that "the majority of mothers do believe their child, with difficult situations and other family stressors occasionally detracting from a mother's willingness to accept the report".

Children who have been abused can feel angry that their mothers did not protect them, and girls can often be angrier with them than with the abuser. This is because they have an ideal of their mothers as all-knowing and all-powerful. Here, again, we see the (arguably) unreal expectations which are placed upon mothers, seen in an idealised way, in this instance by their children.

While most women do exercise those responsibilities which society expects of them – and which they expect of themselves – they may have problems in fully exercising them. What they can do may be inhibited by a lack of material resources and by a sense of powerlessness in their relationship with their partner.

Practical burdens will also fall on a mother following disclosure. Due to the offence, her partner may not be able to work; the woman may have to work to be the breadwinner, but she may also do so to escape from home. Contrarily, she may give up work – and so become socially isolated – because she cannot trust her husband to be alone with their child (supposing that the child has not been taken into care). Support from neighbours and friends, even from family, may drain away or these people even may become actively hostile and statutory agencies may fail to recognise the mother's needs as victim in her own right. Yet the local community may expect more than is usual from a mother in the way of protecting her children. Like Caesar's wife, she must be above suspicion. As one woman told Brogden and Harkin (2000):

> Social services expect you to be their safeguard, their mother ... everything rolled into one but how can you when you are not thinking rationally yourself? You've nobody to talk to. You can't turn round and say to your next door neighbour: "I'm feeling down because ... ". No backing. No support. No nothing. (p. 93)

These authors go so far as to say that

> At the same time as being a victim herself, [she] has to manage the relationship. This management role contains several elements. It means supporting the offender while he goes through a training [presumably a treatment] programme. It involves emotional support. Critically, it requires constant observation of the offender for the sake of her own children. Initially, it can mean ensuring that court appointments are kept. She plays an unpaid role in the justice system.
>
> (Brogden and Harkin 2000: 94)

Protection and blame

The reactions of the public to child sex offenders are usually fairly simple. "Lock them up and throw away the key," "Hanging's too good for them," "Castrate them."

Simplistic public reactions as to how the offender should be treated have their companion in the belief that a mother must, at some level, always have known. This is a belief commonly held. How could she not? Of course, this may be true of some women, but mostly this reaction, too, is one which disregards subtleties when it comes to understanding what a woman knew or didn't know (and what we mean by "know") when it comes to judging a woman's reactions to her partner's actions. Such knowledge is on a continuum, for example, that:

- it is quite possible for abuse to take place and the woman not to know;
- she may be aware that there is something wrong with her child but she is not sure what it is;
- she may know there is something wrong sexually with the relationship but she thinks her partner is having an affair;
- there is an allegation of abuse but the woman doesn't believe it;
- when she finds out, she believes and acts on it immediately;
- she knows about the abuse but redefines the behaviour of the child – "she seems ok";
- the woman knows about the abuse but cannot face the consequences of acknowledging it, since it may involve the loss of the relationship and break-up of family;
- she knows about the abuse but is threatened by her partner;
- she was encouraged to participate in the abuse and did; and
- she participated in the abuse independently of the male offender or in the absence of any partner being present (Wyre 2007).

Hooper and Humphreys (1998) quote their own research (Hooper 1992; Humphreys 1992) to indicate that mothers had a range of "knowledge" about the abuse. Some:

- were totally unaware that abuse was occurring until told by the child or professionals;
- had concerns that "something was wrong" but did not understand what;
- suspected sexual abuse, but were unable to confirm their suspicions (sometimes because their concerns were dismissed by professionals);
- found out that abuse had occurred and believed they had acted protectively, only to find out later that abuse had recurred; and
- spent lengthy periods of time not believing that sexual abuse had occurred, but in time came to realise that it had and subsequently acted protectively. (p. 569)

The reality then stands in complex contrast to the "myths" about mothers as Ovaris (1991) calls them, namely that they:

- knew about the incest and refused to do anything about it;
- were indifferent or absent;
- encouraged their children into incestuous relationships with a father or stepfather;
- wanted their children to "mother" their spouses;
- were weak and submissive;
- kept themselves tired and worn out;

- were frigid; and
- wanted to reverse roles with their daughters. (pp. 1–2)

Thus, the spectrum of knowledge ranges from complete ignorance to partici-pation, with most situations being in between. There is some significance in the use of the terms used to refer to discovery. Professionals talk about "dis-closure", whereas women refer to "finding out". The latter term suggests a more gradual and subtle revelation.

A mother's disbelief at disclosure may be construed as her compliance with, or collusion in the abuse and thus adds to "blame the mother". Disbelief can stem from the revelation of details which are too threatening for her to accept. But even where a woman "knows", there are degrees and ways of knowing and, in knowing, understanding. A woman's knowledge will also be affected by her child's response. How a child reacts to abuse will depend on many factors: the nature and frequency of abuse; how the child perceives it; and who the abuser is. A child may wrongly believe that her mother knows what is happening. In some circumstances there may be only a shadowy under-standing, on the child's part, of what is acceptable and unacceptable behaviour. A child may become withdrawn but also sexualised. Children will very often be sworn to silence by the abuser, whose manipulative ways and general demeanour can also disguise what is happening.

These are not easy signs for a layperson (maybe even many professionals) to read, even if that person is the child's mother. The belief that a mother "must have known" can too easily segue into a belief that she colluded in the abuse or, at very least, that, knowing, she chose not to stop the abuse for any number of reasons. The woman can also be blamed in another way – there was some-thing wrong in her relationship with her partner, something she was unwilling or unable to do, some reaction of which she was incapable, which caused him to act as he did. Had she been a wife in any properly understood sense (whatever that might be) this would not have happened. Or so the argument may go.

Public reactions to women whose children have been abused by a partner must be seen within the context of the long and strong tradition of pointing the finger at mothers when allocating blame for the shortcomings of offspring with regard to all kinds of situations and problems. As Condry (2007) has shown, the long history of mother-blaming has seen mothers made responsible for autism in their children; homosexuality and juvenile delinquency in their sons; and anorexia in their daughters. One study, which she quotes, also found them blamed, in their portrayal in both popular films and academic analyses, for producing serial killers (p. 72). Campbell (1993) found mothers being blamed for riots and unrest on housing estates. The idealisation of motherhood makes for a long fall from grace when child or partner fail to live up to expectations.

Apart from how mother-blaming applies to child sexual abuse, there is generally a greater tolerance in society of men's anti-social behaviour and wrongdoing than that of women. Men are often seen as engaging in "boys will be boys" activities or in the somewhat accepted "that's what men are like" behaviour. When the woman strays, she is seen as failing to accept her responsibilities as wife and mother. Her first call is that of the home; the man's absence from the home is often tolerated, even expected.

Davies and Krane (1996) have shown the extent to which, in child sexual abuse cases, men are not seen as totally accountable because women can be seen as collusive or their perceived "inadequacies" occasioned the abuse. Kelley (1990) showed that social workers, police officers and nurses often made such assumptions. Humphreys (1994: 50) found that the literature of child sexual abuse carried "a legacy of at least 25 years of blaming non-offending mothers either partially or fully for sexual abuse of their children".

All such reactions, knowingly or otherwise, partially shift the responsibility from the abuser to the mother. They make the mother wholly responsible for the child's welfare and protection. It is a very natural thing for any parent to feel that they could have done something to prevent their child being harmed in any way – from an accident in the home to sexual abuse – even when they know rationally that it was impossible for them to have foreseen and prevented the circumstances in which the harm occurred. But with mothers, the burden of expectation creates in them enormous and unjustifiable feelings of guilt when something untoward occurs.

Mothers can fail and are imperfect, but the burden of care, in our society, falls far more heavily upon them. However, mothers are not all alike, even within the same social class. And just as one woman is different from the next, so, too, do offenders differ. It is this also which makes a mother's task of protecting more difficult: she has so much to read. A man may have abused many years ago – he could, for example, have offended as a teenager and is now in his 50s, with his own family. (There was a strong likelihood in the past of adolescent offenders dropping out of the view of the criminal justice and welfare systems because of lack of databases.) While the offence has taken place a long while ago, it could be only after many years – even decades – that it comes to light. This may be because it is only as an adult that the victim now chooses to make the allegation. The allegation may be well founded but with no charge resulting (as in the majority of cases) or, if the offender is charged, there may be no conviction. If a conviction is secured, the offender may turn out to have been a persistent (but hitherto unapprehended) offender. Even if the case brings no conviction, there may still be a strong suspicion that the offender has such a history; or he may not have repeated his abusive behaviour.

All offenders present a risk, but some present a greater risk than others. In all cases, the local authority, police and courts need to be concerned about the protective abilities of the non-abusing partner. A local authority will want to know whether a mother can protect her child, and it is easy for her to see their questioning and inquiry as accusatory and, in fact, it may be ("How could you ever have lived with a man who did that?"). However, defining risk is not a science and lacks consistency. In the same way, mothers cannot be expected always to understand the risks that partners, quite unsuspectingly, may pose, or to act consistently, as hindsight would have them do.

Mothers are victims, too

Some women whose children are abused or whose partner abuses other children have themselves been abused or are in fraught relationships. Hooper (1992), for example, found that all of the 15 women in her study experienced some kind of sexual pressure (p. 45) and "none of these women could be said to be in non-coercive relationships". Eight of them had experienced sexual abuse in their own childhood (p. 47). This "could be a resource on which they drew to understand their children's experiences but it could also be an extra source of guilt" (p. 47).

But even this history may not equip some women with much more knowledge about abuse and abusers than the average person. One women to whom I spoke had been abused by her own father, yet despite that she still said that she had always thought of abusers as "dirty old men in macs" until her daughter's abuse at the hands of her partner was revealed. Paedophile is a term too commonly loosely used and the focus on "paedophiles" can lead a woman to believe that her partner is not a child sex offender because his behaviour does not conform to the pattern of a "paedophile" as she understands it.

Hooper (1992) says that women's own wider experience of childhood may influence how their own child's sexual abuse affects them:

> Those women who had most difficulty in resolving their loss were not those who reported being sexually abused themselves, but those who retained idealised images of their childhoods despite accounts which indicated considerable conflict. (p. 48)

However, Egeland *et al.* (1988) found

> that women who were aware of their own past history of abuse and how it has affected them were less likely to have child care problems later than those who were not.

A disproportionate number of mothers whose children have been abused were themselves abused as children (Smith 1994). A woman who has herself suffered in this way is likely to have her distress exacerbated by her child's disclosure (Brickman 1993). This was confirmed by Deblinger *et al.* (1994), who compared the mothers of abused children who had themselves been abused with mothers of abused children who had not. However, the way in which the women reacted to their children did not differ between the two groups. Thus, what is perhaps more significant is the way in which those who had themselves been abused dealt with that abuse, not the fact that they had such a history.

Pat (Mosaic Women Writers' Group no date) writes:

> It was while I was getting counselling ... that it brought to a head my own childhood experiences which wasn't about sexual but mental abuse,

watching my mother and father fighting and then weeks and weeks of silence in the house. It brought all that to a head. I also started to deal with the feelings I had about myself as well as the feelings I had about what had been done to my daughter. It would all come out muddled, my daughter and me, a bit of my daughter, a bit of me.

A woman's history of abuse is only one part of her life. She also plays many other roles: wife, girlfriend, lover, mother, daughter, employer, employee, neighbour. But, when an allegation is made, all aspects of her life are exposed to family and public scrutiny. This makes sexual abuse and its repercussions for those closest to the offender a unique crime. All serious crime presents problems for partners and families but no other not even rape, routinely breaks open for public view the intimacies of a relationship and the details of an (innocent) partner's life. The sexual abuse of children brings with it connotations and shadows that lurk in our psyche – about the offender, about his partner, indeed, about ourselves. Thus, a woman wanting to rebuild her life may find that difficult to do; the paths will be closed or obscured. This will be the more so if she chooses to try and rebuild that life by taking her partner back into the home.

A man may have sexually abused a child in the family, but his behaviour will have had a harmful impact on others in the family and on the family generally. Thus, it is important that partners (and non-abused) children are recognised as secondary victims. For a man who is taken into custody and then sentenced to a long term of imprisonment (although this will not happen to the majority of offenders), it may mean that he has not had to face his family or neighbours once the arrest took place. But his partner finds herself living in the same community, seeing the same people each day, attending family events as in the past. Alternatively, she may be forced to move away from a familiar place, where she may have had formerly supportive relationships. She may even, in extreme cases, have to break with her family and her partner's family.

Secondary victimhood may be experienced in various ways. There are many, various and continuing losses that a woman faces when her child is abused and these may be more extensive when her partner is the abuser (Hooper 1992). A loss of attachment maybe experienced as a loss of self. There is a loss of trust. If the partner goes to prison, is removed from the home, and/or the relationship breaks up, there is the loss of that relationship and, with it, the attendant losses of income and maybe even home. Should the child go into care, there is the loss of the child and the loss of the family unit. There may be loss of identity as a good and protective mother and (where the partner favoured the child over the woman) loss of her sense of attractiveness or femininity. All of this may also create a sense loss of purpose in life.

A mother is distraught at what has befallen her child; she has been betrayed by someone whom she may have loved and trusted; and she may well face the obloquy of the community. A woman who takes her partner back may seem to confirm what neighbours and family may have felt – either that she "knew", that she colluded in the abuse, or that she was less than vigilant about her child's safety. Neighbourly disapproval may come in the form of verbal abuse, but extreme cases of violence against women have been reported. Brogden and Harkin (2000: 94) recount a case, in Northern Ireland, where the family home was destroyed by fire. Testimonies in this book include those of women who have had to leave their family homes (in one case a woman has changed her name) and, as reported above, one woman returned to her home to collect some clothes, after being taken to a women's refuge, to find that neighbours had stolen from her home what they could not destroy.

The initial shock and sheer disbelief that women experience can be, literally, traumatic. They can experience exclusion and rejection, failure and shame. They may blame themselves. They may be blamed by the community, either as surrogates for what their partner did, or because of the suspicion that "she must have known" and was thus, in some way, party to what happened. A woman who was helped by the Parents for Protection programme said that she was told that hers was now "an abused family", when disclosure was made, a description she found "apt".

Another woman, at the same project, wrote that the "sentence" she and her child received was a life-long one (Mosaic Women Writers' Group no date). One woman, whose husband received six months in prison suspended for two years, wrote: "We got a life sentence" (Anonymous 1994). Brogden and Harkin (2000: 89) describe being the partner of an abuser as "a pretty tough lifetime assignment". One mother said how she was "eaten up with so much guilt and horror that this had happened to them [her children]". But she felt that at least now they could sleep without fear, with their door open. Yet she reports her child saying to her:

> "Mommy, I feel sorry for you." I says: "You feel sorry for me. It's you that have been through everything" and she says: "No. My hell is over. Your hell is starting".
>
> (Brogden and Harkin 2000: 91)

The same authors were told by a man who had abused someone else's child but whose partner had had to move to a hostel: "Your own family is a victim" (p. 92).

Not surprisingly, a very high percentage of women whose children have been abused suffer from depression. When abuse is within the family this tends to be less (50 per cent) than when the abuse occurs outside of the family (69 per cent) (Wagner 1991). Less common are suicide attempts, although the figures are still high. In a study of 201 families, Goodwin (1981) found that there were 11 (5.4 per cent) suicide attempts. Within these 11 families there were 13 attempts, 5 by mothers and 8 by daughters who were the direct victims of abuse.

A mother can lose her children to care as result of disclosure where, for example, she chooses to reunite with a man whom the local authority regards as unsafe and where it believes the mother cannot protect the child. However,

Pellegrin and Wagner (1990) found that among the two most significant factors in professionals' decisions about removing the child from the home were a mother's willingness to believe her child and a mother's cooperation with agencies. These were more significant than how frequent and severe was the abuse. Mothers' perceived ability and willingness to protect children from further abuse is also crucial in this regard (p. 4). How mothers respond to disclosure is also critical to children's recovery.

The mother as protector of her child and other children

While the majority of perpetrators are men, the task of protection, as stated above, falls largely on women. Hooper (1992) concludes from various studies that a higher number of incidents are disclosed to mothers than to outside agencies and that the less girls are able to protect themselves, the more they are likely to turn to their mothers than to their friends. (Boys are less likely to tell anyone). "The bulk of the work of child protection is done not by professionals but by children themselves, their friends and parents," she writes (Hooper 1992: 2).

This is something very rarely acknowledged, especially in the professional literature. Thus, it is important to emphasise that all women should be able to protect their children, and this remains the case even where the offence causes the relationship to end. But women can also play a vital part in protecting other children where the relationship continues. Brogden and Harkin (2000) state:

> Monitoring behaviour, as well as complicity, is best conducted by the nearest and dearest. If an offender is not to re-offend, a partner to whom obligations are tight and who can withdraw affection as a sanction, is crucial. The survival of such a partnership might be crucial to prevent re-offending. (p. 92)

These authors also say that, "given the low *recorded* rates of re-offending by incest abusers, one success story may lie within that community observation and informal control" (p. 86).

In fact, little attention by politicians, policy makers and those providing services is given to informal methods, and this was even more so before the creation of Circles of Support and Accountability and Stop It Now! (see Chapter 3). The law and professionals, like social workers and probation officers, are seen as being the agents of surveillance and control of ex-offenders. This has tended to lead to the community and, especially, the family being ignored for this purpose. Yet those closest to the ex-offender are best placed both to observe him and to impose sanctions and express disapproval for any inappropriate behaviour.

A stable lifestyle – a job, housing and so on – is assumed to equate with a low reconviction rate and so, "nowhere is that stability in social control more important than in [the] spousal relationship" (Brogden and Harkin 2000: 86). These authors interviewed 27 abusers, as well as drawing on testimonies from agency staff and partners. They say: "There is no equivalent of an AA meeting for abusers. An intimate was crucial to reinforcing the lessons of the treatment programme" (p. 87). However, since then the Sexual Behaviour Unit and Mosaic in Newcastle-upon-Tyne have combined to create support and monitoring groups for men who either have historic convictions for sexual abuse but who are now outside of the criminal justice system, or have never been convicted. It is likely that these groups are unique.

Ex-offenders, whatever risk they are believed to pose, can all find themselves in a high-risk situation of another sort: the high risk that they will be suspected of doing something that they have not done. Thus, a partner's backing, say Brogden and Harkin (2000), is necessary to allay suspicion, for her mere presence – at the shops, on the school run, out and about generally – avoids unjustifiable accusation.

For a woman to adopt such a role – especially given all she and her children will have suffered as a result of the offence, even if the abuse was not within the family – requires great resilience and commitment. What she offers is company in the midst of social isolation; security against mistaken suspicion; emotional support when the offender is depressed; and support during any treatment programme.

A life apart

A woman's decision to separate from her partner may be influenced by factors other than the abuse he has committed. None of the 15 women interviewed by Hooper (1992), for example, decided to separate from her partner on the basis of the abuse alone.

Middle-class women may enjoy more financial security than working-class women, even when both are in paid jobs. If middle-class women are not working, but divorced, they may be cushioned by a financial settlement, although none of the women to whom Hooper (1992) spoke complained of financial hardship, even though several of them were on benefits. Middle-class women fear the stigma of contact with statutory agencies; working-class women fear the loss of their children. (This is not to say that middle-class women do not *also* fear the loss of their children, but they are not so used to contact with statutory agencies as many working-class women may be. Such agencies are they often regarded not as helpful and supportive but as policing and threatening.) Older women, who have been dependent on their partners, have less chance of getting a job; for younger women, the prospects may be better. Younger women may have higher expectations of their marriages or believe that the prospect of a new partner is likely; older women may see little hope of a new relationship (Hooper 1992).

Any woman who is a single parent has a tougher job in so many ways – in terms of raising her children, materially and socially – than a woman in a relationship, but for a woman who is single because the offending of her partner has forced this on her all this is exacerbated.

As has been said, women whose partners sexually abuse children are victims who have suffered emotionally, and in many other ways. They have the burdens of child protection and of policing the offender placed on them if he returns to the family home, as well costs to their material welfare and that of their child (but they may also suffer if he doesn't). They often pay a cost in terms of social disapproval. Their needs are many, but they are rarely met. They suffer, literally, in silence. They often carry all of these burdens unaided.

But knowing that others are in the same situation is something that can help them, and being able (though this is rarely possible) to meet with them and share experiences can be a lifeline, as Pat so eloquently records in her experience of the Partners for Protection programme:

> I don't think I would ever have coped or come to terms with my feelings, I don't think I would have been able to do anything logical with my thoughts and feelings. I needed to talk to mothers who had experienced the same thing. They understood everything, all my feelings, and I think everything I blurted out, upside down or what; other mothers understood exactly as I felt. It wouldn't have been good talking to even a really close friend; I tried that and they were very sympathetic but you just knew they didn't have that connection, that same experience. I mean you could talk to a perfect stranger and that really helped, you knew they really understood. It was easier to talk to someone like that than someone really close to you; they would try and understand, be very sympathetic, but really didn't know how you felt. It was talking to the other mothers, I could talk to these mothers really easily, it was like I had been with these people all my life even though I didn't know them.
>
> (Mosaic Woman Writers' Group no date)

The Women's Stories

Chris Roberts

"You don't know what they're thinking and they're secretly blaming you"

Chris Roberts is 45 and was abused by her father from the age of 11 until she was 30. He had suffered from mental illness. Ten years ago, as a single mother, she met a man of the same age, Sean Francis. At the time he was under investigation for an offence against his step-grandchild for which, eventually, he was never charged. It is believed that he may have sexually abused three other step-grandchildren and a niece. Chris and Francis had a daughter, Chantelle, who, it is believed, he began abusing when she was 3. She is now 9, and has been diagnosed as having moderate learning disabilities and behavioural problems. She attends a special school. Arrested, Francis was never charged with any offence against her. Chris's eldest daughter, 26-year-old Carol, has a 2-year-old son. Chris uses a Zimmer frame and her arms show the scars where she has harmed herself. She suffers from depression, panic attacks, and has a history of mental illness and is physically disabled.

He was somebody I had known for 20-odd year; me best mate was Di, his sister-in-law. Dee, her lassie, used to go and stay with him and his wife every weekend from when she was, like, two year old, so it was the least thing on me mind ever thinking that he would ever do anything like that. He came to where I was staying, which was just up the street from his sister-in-law, when he come to the village. He told us all what he had been accused of. He said that Kylie, his step-granddaughter, had stepped over the camera that he had rigged up to the telly, which had fallen on the floor – he was an alarm engineer – and she told her mamme she saw her bummie on the telly. Of course, straight away the mam went running over. "What the hell's going on?" and he explained what he had said and then he was arrested. He said that the reason Cath, his wife, was pushing it was because she wanted him out of the way so she could get all her stuff out of the house. His wife had wanted to leave him but was frightened to leave him so she concocted this story with her daughters, who never liked him to start with, so he was arrested, and while he was locked up for the weekend they cleared the house.

Cath told the neighbours and everything, so he had to leave Newcastle where he was from. He come down and he seen his sister-in-law and she said that he could stay there. 'Course she didn't believe it, and as I had known him and his sister-in-law for a lot of years, I was willing to believe what she, you know, thought best and, as I say, I knew that her bairn had stopped every weekend from the age of two.

Di said that he could move in with her. Now his two stepdaughters both had husbands and they come down looking for him. They knew where Di lived but they didn't know nothing about me, so I says to Di, when they landed at her door threatening, "He can come and stop with us, me and me daughter Carol, because they don't know where I live. He can sleep in Carol's bedroom and Carol will just sleep in with me." So we agreed and it went like that for three months, we were like that, just platonic, and then after the three months we started a relationship. Of course, the first time I slept with him, I fell pregnant, and that was me daughter Chantelle who he eventually abuses.

Everything about what he did with Kylie was reported to the police but I didn't know that, though. He didn't let on that there was any charges, but anyway social services become involved with me. All they said was they believed he could be a risk to me daughter [Carol] because she was only 14 at the time. But anytime social services come to the house and if they said anything, he would go storming down to the office, you know, really making it look as if he was innocent. He told all me friends what he had been accused of, they sided with him; he didn't hide it from nobody. I was in denial all the way. I had a lot of mental health problems. I was on a lot of medication so I was very vulnerable and (obviously learnt through the [Partners for Protection] course) that's the sort of people that they [child sex offenders] go for. Anyway, social services were involved and then all of a sudden they stopped.

He was knocking around with Roy, a lad who lived at the top of the estate, because he was into computers the same as he was. Then the lad's daughter, Suzie, made an allegation against her father saying that he had been touching her. For some unknown reason her mam asked her for to draw a picture of what her dad looked like down below and because the bairn drew a picture and put hair around it, her mam gave her a good hiding and said she was a liar because apparently he always shaved down there, but on past experience of what I've learnt about me ex-partner, he never did anything by hisel', he always made sure there was two of them, him and another one. That's where it knackered me case up because he was knocking around with somebody who had been accused of the same thing so they couldn't prove who had done it.

I was so naive then about paedophiles, I didn't know nothing about them apart from what they did, but as far as we had been brought up, they were little old men in dirty macs; that's that way we portray it. This man [Francis] was a big stocky lad, he used to be a bouncer on the doors, you know what I mean? The neighbours used to say you could never meet a nicer bloke. I didn't believe it because I thought it was just Cath's way of getting him out of the way so she could leave. I knew their marriage was rocky, they where always arguing and stuff like that, so I just didn't think he could do something like that.

I thought we were happy: we didn't really even argue very much. He just got on with his computers, but when I look back it was like he was all for knocking around with younger kids – not people his own age (one laddie,

Mick, he was 16). Looking back, he intimidated them. I think it was a power thing because the kids obviously wouldn't answer him back. He would take them up to the town with him and that and go shoplifting. He didn't have a job and I don't know where the money came from. I never seen it, I never ever seen it. We had income support. He claimed for me and for the bairn.

When Chantelle was born, he was very protective. From the day he found out that I was pregnant, he said it was going to be a little girl and she was going be called Chantelle and it wasn't until I actually did the protection course that it dawned on us that Chantelle is "shan't tell, she shan't tell anybody". Yes, he had it planned all the time. He knew exactly what he was doing. It was digital penetration. We believe she was three when it started but it wouldn't have been very long, just a matter of months. Social services had disappeared off the scene for nearly two year but they come back on the scene and they said that they were still saying that they thought he posed a risk to me daughter Chantelle. So I says – me temper was getting up by this time – I says, "If you're so bloody sure that he's done something, we'll get the bairn checked." He was very upset and he says, "She's not going, she's not going. I've never touched her. You're not putting me bairn through that," so we sort of like did it on the quiet. He went down to the social services, he was bawling and shouting and he got asked to leave the premises or they we going to call the police.

So we made an appointment, went to the hospital, got her checked. The doctor came in, she spoke to us first then told the bairn she was going examine her, you know, down below and not to be frightened, she was a doctor, it was all right for a doctor, so I was just holding her hand when she examined her. Then she said she needed to see another doctor to come and have a look so another doctor came and had a look and they both agreed that her hymen was broken and she had been sexually abused so they started taking photographs of the bairn down below with a special camera that they use.

God! Whack! It was like somebody had kicked us straight in the face when they come back and said she had been sexually abused. I was gutted – I just couldn't take it in, I couldn't take it in at all, and then for to have to wait a week for them to get their information together which was – oh! – I cannot describe it. I had been in denial and he had … the five year we were together – it had all been a lie, everything about it had been a lie, and he had used me to have a child that he could abuse.

I got the bairn ready, went back outside where the social worker was and they said I had to call the police in. They came to see me the same day. I was round at a friend's and they asked me if I would keep it to meself until they got all their evidence together so that they could get him and there was no way he could wangle out of it, so I agreed to that, not knowing it was going take them over a week, so for a week I had to live with him and pretend that everything was all right, knowing what he had done to the bairn.

I'm on a lot of medication for me nerves to start with, always have been since '94, so I just made out that I was ill and, well, it didn't take much making out – I was! I was in bed a lot by this time, the bairn was in temporary foster care. He knew that I knew about his past by this time and I says that they were saying that he posed a risk to the bairn. He says, "Well, what happened at the medical?" I says, "I've got to wait, they're going to let us know."

We were supposed to have a meeting with social services. He went to the meeting with the bairn without telling me, he just said he was going out for a walk with her and then social services had said to him that I had to be there so he come back up, because it wasn't far from our house. He come back up and he said, "Social services just want to see we all." I said, "What do you mean?" He says, "Well, they have kicked all this clart [fuss] off. They're saying that I'm posing a risk to the bairn", and he started crying. He says, "They're going to take her off we." I says, "What for? We've done nothing wrong." So we went down and they had two police standing outside. We went in and they said he posed a high risk to the bairn and they wanted me to sign her into temporary foster care for her safety. By this time I was a complete and utter wreck, but they were just talking to me at the time. They made me sign the temporary foster care papers. In the meantime he had walked out of the building, past the two policemen with the bairn and he did off and they couldn't find him, so they come and told me that he had legged it with the bairn and could I think of anywhere he could have went to. The only place I could think of was our friends at the time, Karen and Steve, and they lived just round the corner from us. Steve answered the door, said he hadn't seen him and then eventually it worked out he was there anyway, so he came out and they brought him back in the police car with the bairn. He was sent off on his merry way and I was taken with the bairn to the placement for her, temporary foster placement.

When the neighbours found out … he went round and told them because obviously they had seen the police, he told them that the police had arrested me for neglect on the bairn and that was why the police had come to the house with me. But it wasn't, it was the police and the social worker taking me to the house to get some of me clothes because all I had was what I was standing in and then they were taking me to a women's refuge.

I'd been to the women's refuge and then me friend and the social worker took me over to the house. By that time I had been told the house had been smashed up, but I never expected nothing like it was. When the neighbours found out what had really happened, they smashed up me house completely, I mean there was nothing left. When I was in the refuge they stole everything out of me kitchen – me cooker, me fridge freezer, every single thing … the washer – everything electrical out of the kitchen, they stole. What they couldn't steal, they destroyed and they told me friend – because she found out who they were – that the reason that they had done it was to get at him. She says, "You knew that Chris was coming back to that house once he was arrested." Just to get at him! Why did they take the bairn's collection of porcelain dolls? I went back expecting to pick some of me things up that were treasured possessions that I had from me bairn's being little. They had even slashed the wallpaper on the walls, me kitchen ceiling was on the floor because what they couldn't pinch and what they couldn't smash, they flooded the place, they burst main pipes upstairs and flooded the place. I had (well, it was his) it was like a cockatiel and that was lying dead in its cage, obviously it had drowned. The council workers had put shutters on the front of the house but they hadn't put them on the back so, of course, they just kicked the back door in, but nobody seen nothing. How they got all that furniture out without anybody seeing anything? It's just … I can't believe nobody's seen nothing.

Everything, just everything was smashed. I had had this painting, it is painted on glass but I've had it 20 odd year. I bought it when I was pregnant with me oldest daughter and that, and the portrait of me two bairns together, was the only few things in the house that wasn't smashed, so I knew it had to be somebody who knew me and it turned out it was me next-door neighbour. Him and his sister-in-law had went in when they were pie-eyed and done it. They smashed up but they didn't steal anything, they just smashed the place. It was others that broke in the back and stole.

I went into the women's refuge, I went into a B&B for one night, then I was placed into the women's refuge in Howden. Then a few weeks' later, he was arrested. The police came and arrested him after the week I had been making out that nothing was wrong. He started saying, "I haven't done nothing, Christine. I didn't touch her, I didn't touch her, I swear I didn't, I didn't". I just stood there and just looked at him, I wanted to pick up a knife and stab him, that's how … I was mixed up so much. The police took him away.

I was in the women's refuge for nine months, I was getting regular contact with me bairn twice a week, I was seeing her with the social worker. It was supervised all the time right up until just before she come back home. I had umpteen different social workers because they couldn't place a certain one because they were stretched to their limit. The social worker that I had had a filing system that was a cardboard box, so you can imagine what sort of time I went through with him. For something that me and the bairn had just been through, to give us a male social worker I thought was all wrong.

We started to go to court, because he started fighting us for custody, and he wanted having access with the bairn. Social services turned round and said, "Could we give him indirect contact with the bairn?" I says, "What does that mean?", she says, "Well, we'll write to him every so often and let him know how she is getting on." I says, "Don't say another word – do you think for one fucking – excuse me – minute, one fucking minute, I am going to let you tell him how she is doing and him find out how he has wrecked our lives?"

Me bairn's now in a special school, she's stuck in the mind of a 3-year-old, she has got no sense of danger, got no modesty whatsoever. She has … we don't know if it's eczema or psoriasis, but the doctor says it's stress-related and every now and again it flares up. I fought for two and a half year to get the bairn back. The last two court appearances went a bit south: they tried to get him for what he had done but because the bairn was under the age of 6, she was too young to be a witness because she wouldn't possibly be able to relay the right story. She has the mind of a 3-year-old, and because the bairn couldn't relay the same story twice they labelled her a liar. I have actually got the police report of what that bairn said had happened and how they could not convict him on that bairn's statement I will never, till this day, know.

I couldn't even get him for "finding of fact" [whereby a judge decides if abuse has occurred based on the information available], which meant that if he went into another family they would be able to go in and tell the other family what he had been accused of which obviously they couldn't with me because he has got all this human rights. The child protection officer that was dealing with me – big burly bloke, he was massive – he actually cried. He was punching his own car when he had to tell me that they wouldn't even take the case into court; he just couldn't believe it. He said, "I just don't even know how to tell you". I says, "Quick and fast, as quick as you can, just tell us." He said, "They'll not take it into court because he was knocking around with that Roy at the time and he had been accused of sexual abuse so they can't prove who it was. It could have been him [Roy] that was abusing her."

Chantelle went into foster care because I failed to protect her but I thought, at first, that it was unfair. How was I supposed to know? I was on a lot of medication, but he used to make sure I took me medication and that I took the right ones and it was actually two year after that I seen the same social worker, and I was away from him by this time, and she couldn't believe it was the same person she was talking to. It was actually her that said has he been drugging me with me medication? It's possible because it's never happened since I've been away from him.

Naturally, you think what are they [social services] thinking? They wanted me to sort of admit that I had failed to protect Chantelle and that was when Mosaic come into it. Social services were all up ready for adoption with Chantelle until I seen Professor [Don] Grubin [director of the Sexual Behaviour Unit] – he was American – and he said that I deserved the chance to do the protection course.

It was unbelievable, unbelievable the things that we learnt. As I said before, I was of the understanding that a paedophile was a little old man in a dirty mac. You know in them days when I was young, it was. We learnt not to judge each other as well [on the course]. There was some of the lasses there who, even though they knew what their husbands had done to their children they still wanted to be with them and keep their children, and we learnt not to judge them. We were all there for a reason, we weren't there to condemn each other, and I actually wrote a short life story of me life. I never thought of me life because I was abused as a child off me father and it was sort of like … we were supposed to write a short paragraph about our lives because we used to get homework, and I ended up writing 41 pages on A4-sized paper. I did a couple of poems.

But me and another lass were the only two out of the whole group that got our bairns back, but I fought for two and a half year to get Chantelle and to stop him from seeing her. I had a heart attack in the meantime through the stress of the court case. Then the last two hearings the judge was rather pee'd off because he [Francis] didn't attend, he had given his solicitor no grounds of what to work on, so his solicitor was pee'd off because he was standing there looking a right idiot. The judge gave me an order which meant that if he applied to the courts for to get access it would be just thrown out. Usually they just give you it for a couple of year, well they gave me it till she's 18, so if he goes to court in the meantime to get access, it will just be thrown out.

He's in jail now, but not for what he's done to Chantelle. [She produces a newspaper cutting from an envelope in her bag about her ex-partner's case and his conviction and jailing for two and a half years on 12 charges, including threats to kill, racially aggravated harassment, causing fear of violence by making threatening telephone calls while working as a security guard.] It's at the end [of the newspaper report] where they say about him not doing this sort of thing again, I actually wanted to go to the *Evening Chronicle* and tell them me story. I asked one of the lasses here [at the course], and she said they wouldn't touch it because he could probably sue them.

[Of the newspaper cutting] It's a reminder, it's sort of … I don't know … it's, like, it makes me feel better knowing that he's in jail. I mean I feel sorry for what he's done, the people he's done it to, but it's me little bit of justice. I'm getting some justice for what he's done to the bairn. But I got him sent down for six months for threats to kill on me social worker and the health visitor. He said he was going to put a bomb under their car, as if he would know how to make one!

Chantelle's in temporary foster care again at the minute because of me health. We are having a lot of trouble with me chest and me back, but it's only temporary. I'm highly depressed, anxiety, panic attacks, me spine's compressing, I've got arthritis in both me knees, I've got arthritis in both me hands, I've got tennis elbow through exercising trying to lose the weight; just loads and loads of things. I have angina now. But I have her Fridays, Saturdays and Sundays. She's in a special school. She's 9, she can't even write, even copying, she can't even write the letter "A". She knows that her name begins with a "C". She's got moderate learning disabilities, behavioural problems, she's got no concentration, lack of concentration. She is getting a lot better now from what she was since she has went to the special school. Of course, the foster mum's the Wicked Witch of the West because she gets made to go to bed at eight and when she is with me, well it's a weekend, she's not at school so she is allowed to stay up a little bit later.

She is so, so loving but she will be loving to anybody and she tries to mother me, you know. She knows the reason she's in temporary foster care is because of me ill-health and with them telling her that she tries to mother us, because she thinks if she makes me better then she will get to come back home. She doesn't understand the proper context of what's going on.

I had a real bad experience with the social worker who has now just been changed. She actually arranged to meet me and I thought it was just for a quick chat. She arranged to meet me at McDonald's and, as we were sitting there, she told me that they were going to look for a long-term placement for Chantelle because with the short-term placement she was in, it was taking me longer for to get better than what they had expected, so they can't keep shuffling her about in case I am still not well after the next short-time placement.

I said, "How long is long term?", and she says, "How long's a piece of string?", and I says, "Well, what are we looking at, what are we talking about?" She says, "You know they always come back in the end." I says, "When's that? When she's 18?" She says, "You know the score," and she told me all this sitting in McDonald's and, of course, you can imagine the state I was in. I went and seen the solicitor and told the solicitor what it had went in McDonald's and she wrote to social services' legal department and ever since then the social worker has been on the sick. Now she's wrote me a letter saying she didn't know how long she was going to be off, so she was assigning her case over to somebody else so I wasn't just keep getting every willy-nilly who was free so I have got a new social worker now who really seems nice.

The lass [foster parent] that's got her now, I mean, she's 60. She's had heart problems so if she lifts up something too heavy her back could go, and she will be in a wheelchair for the rest of her life. This is where I struggle to under-stand how somebody with this many problems as what I've got can look after her and they're saying that I couldn't manage her on a weekend without the home help I have come in. They come for an hour on a night time to help bath Chantelle and then they just play with her, you know, calm her down for bed.

We play things like "Frustration" and do craft. She loves her craft work, she is very good at that and computers. She's very quick with her computers and she has actually won two medals for gymnastics – for the floor and the vault – and she won the competition to represent the region. Her class won that so they went up to Durham to the competition and she come back with a silver and a bronze. She can't be left outside to play by herself. None of the other kids bother with her. There was one mother I actually overheard saying to her daughter that she wasn't allowed to play with Chantelle because she wasn't right in the head, just nasty, nasty talk like that.

She's seen a doctor and she was only in the room five minutes and he says, "The child's wearing me out", but I think it's now we are going to have to start looking at some form of help. She does play therapy in school where she's allowed to express any sort of feelings. She can even swear. She knows that outside that room she's not allowed to, but she will tell you, she'll say, "I can even say the 'f' word". She will not sleep with her bedroom door shut, she's got to have some light, well they're just like fairy lights I've got up on her wall, she has got to have them on.

There was one time she talked about what happened. She says that he had tried to make her bummie bleed: there was no evidence on like her back pas-sage being touched, there was just her vagina. She talks about "the long time ago house" [where the family used to live] but then she'll say something that never ever happened, but to her mind I think it's her way of coping. She said that her daddy was on the roof and he fell off and he smashed his head open and she'll give such an evil little laugh at the end of it, as if she's really pleased that it's happened. It never did happen but she will tell you the same story over and over again and I think that's her way of coping.

She was having really bad nightmares when she was first in foster care. The foster carer would find her asleep behind the settee or behind the bedroom door. She was curled up in a little ball outside the foster carer's door when she was getting up in the morning. She had actually found her asleep on the toilet floor. She had obviously wet herself; she was soaking wet. She used to scream out at night. She'll not have the door shut because she tells you that "in the long time ago house" daddy broke her door and she had tried to stop him from getting in and he had pushed. He didn't break the door. I don't know if he's pushed it and she's been against the door or what. At that age I don't think she would comprehend.

I started to notice, because she was still in nappies, that her nappies were on the wrong way but bairns do all that you know, they take their nappies off – they're just disposable nappies – they pull them off and all this, but now thinking back I know there was a few times her nappy had been interfered with.

Just like when she used to cry. He used to like to send me to the bingo every night. It was supposed it was our last £20 and he would say "Go on, get yourself to the bingo," and I used to go off tappy lapping [happily] to the bingo and it was then that he was getting at the bairn. He was getting me out the way and when he couldn't get me out the way he was drugging me so I was asleep. Me next door neighbour used to hear the bairn crying but then she would hear them laughing she just thought the bairn had been naughty and had been told off. Now, to this day she just can't believe what was actually going on.

I can't trust anybody. I have been on me own ever since. I'll not let a man in the house. When me oldest daughter came back to live, she used to have her friends in and, of course, I got to know them as they were coming in and that. She had one friend who was a lot older than her and they would be sitting up all night blinkin' watching films and talking and stuff.

I had made me bedroom a safety net: if I felt panic attacks coming on, I would go into me bedroom because no man had ever been in the room. One night I shouted down for them to turn the music down and he come running up the stairs: "Hello, mam!" He come straight in me bedroom and that was it. I just lost all security in me bedroom, I mean I practically hoyed him down the stairs. He was just, you know, saying, "Hello, mam, are you alright? Are you not coming down?" but it just knocked me and now I've got nowhere I can call safe in me house. I don't feel safe in it no more because there's a man been up the stairs. I promised the bairn that no man would ever, ever go up the stairs because she was frightened on a night time.

Me oldest one, Carol, she is getting married in April [2008]. She's got a little son who will be 2 in January, proper little corker he is. Chantelle's going to be bridesmaid so she's really looking forward to that.

Carol just lived her own life basically. She went to live with her boyfriend when she was nearly 16 – it was just across the road – but she hated him. She was 3 year old when I left him [Carol's father]. He had access to come and see her but he was an alcoholic and he mucked his access up. I got a letter off the social security, the job centre, saying that he was now in work and he was going to start paying maintenance and would I let them know when I got payment. I'm still waiting for it, yet and I have never had another letter off the social security asking why I haven't informed them about these payments. Me father chased him away from the door one day because he had missed his week that he was supposed to come [to see Carol] so he thought he could just turn up the next one.

I was abused meself by me father till I was a woman – nearly 30. The first time that it happened, I just couldn't believe it had happened. I thought it had been a nightmare. It was just touching till he thingied hiself off. It was, like, every Friday. I used to go out on a Friday. You get all dolled up and you're going to the club. That was the only night of the week I used to go out and, I don't know, with being all dolled up and that I don't know what was going through his mind but I worked it out when he first abused me. That was when me father had become mentally ill. He had just touched me on the chest, wey, I mean, there was nowt there! I was only 11. That's where I think me mental illness has come from.

He was back and forward seeing specialists. He died when Chantelle was only months old, but he never ever touched Carol, even when we were living in the same house as him, and that was why I didn't kick up a fuss as much, or tell anybody. I kept it hidden because as long as I knew he was touching me I knew he wasn't touching her. You know what I mean – I sort of, in a way, allowed it as long as I knew he wouldn't touch her. Me mam didn't know about it until I cracked up in '94. I had a mental breakdown and I ended up in St George's [a local hospital] and that's when it all come out, but they didn't believe it. I've got two brothers, one older, one younger. It was all brushed under the carpet. For me mam's sake, I'll not bring it up. They still to this day don't believe it. There's a lot of things I could have said but I didn't want to hurt me mam, who's in her 70s now but she's fitter than me. I keep saying to meself, "God forbid when me mam goes, I'm going to tell them and make them understand," but I don't think I ever will; I think it's just this thing of wanting to know that they believe that I wouldn't make up such a thing as that. I mean, how could they think I would be so wicked, that I would make up something like that? When it happened with Chantelle, me oldest brother I never really heard from, me youngest brother he was up in arms. Well, I'm saying me oldest brother wasn't sort of like acknowledging, but the two of them wanted to go and gan him a good hiding, but what's the use of that?

Why's it repeating itself? What the hell have I done that was so wrong that I should have to go through this, with Chantelle? I went through a time where I actually went shoplifting just so I could get caught, just so I could punish meself because nobody had been punished for what had happened to the bairn. Somebody had to be punished and because I couldn't punish him, I was punishing meself. I still am to this day, punishing meself, not through shoplifting – I've stopped all that – but the guilt. Now it's nervous pricking: I've got scars all over. I'll just sit and gouge, I cannot stop it; sometimes I don't even know I'm doing it.

I'm seeing a counsellor now. The last one that I used to see was a CPN [community psychiatric nurse]. I couldn't really talk to her. I couldn't really tell everything that had actually went on because I felt so ashamed, I felt like a prostitute, I suppose, that I was wasn't one, that I wasn't getting paid. I don't know, I couldn't connect with her and then I started seeing another one and it was like they wanted more to concentrate on what was happening now than what had happened in the past, and it's what's happened in the past that's reflecting now, so I need to go through it all. It's no good saying, "We'll concentrate on what's happening now, the past is the past, put it away, put it in a box and lock it." It's no good: I've got to live it and I've got to tell it all, every little detail for to get it out, so I can start putting it into place, and understand why it happened, it's still …

I know how it works, I know how they [sex offenders] groom you. They have got their four obstacles [to overcome] before they actually do anything, but it's still up here [she taps her forehead] the way I dealt with it at the time and how I think I should have dealt with it, how I should have noticed things and didn't notice them. Now I would notice straight away because of the eight weeks that I done with [the Partners for Protection course] it's just, like, I don't trust any bloke at all that's tried to get close or even just trying to be a friend. I couldn't … I mean, I trust you because I know what your job is and that you are trying to help the likes of people like us, but …

The aftermath of what's happened, it doesn't just stop there once they're locked up. We live with it for the rest of our lives, they get punished for so many years. The police were never even involved with me dad. I went to his funeral when he died but I've never cried, I never cried the day I was told that he had died. He was cutting his toe nails when it happened, he went just like that, it was an aneurism. He wasn't ill, he had his depression and that's how I've coped with most of what he done, through making meself believe it was because he was ill at the time, knowing what I'm going through and seeing similarities in the way me depression goes on to the way his went on. I try to understand, make excuses for him really. I suppose that's how I've coped with some of that by keep telling meself that it wasn't me real dad [because he was mentally ill] that was like that, me real dad wouldn't have been like that, you know. But the bairn's father: I just cannot wait till he's six feet under. I would go to his funeral just to make sure he was buried and that would be the only reason.

Me mam rarely talked about it. Me mam's a very close, deep person; she keeps things to herself, you don't know exactly how she's coping with it because she'll not talk openly about it. She is a loving grandma to the bairn, you know, but me mam's more firmer with her than what I am because I feel so guilty that it was me fault that things have happened to her. I'll never ever get rid of that guilt and I'll never ever stop blaming meself for what's happened to her but that's something I've got to try and live with.

I don't think me mam ever liked me ex. She used to put on a face – all mother-in-laws do – but he had a face for her and her only, where he was such a good son-in-law. She never let on. If she wanted something done she wouldn't, even if we were sitting there, have turned round and asked him to do it. She would rather wait until me brother or me nephew, who is grown up now, came and she would ask them to do it. She was never beholden to him for anything. She's never turned round and says that it was me bloody fault or how didn't you see what was going on. She's never put blame, but I think sometimes that can be worse than actually being blamed, because you don't know what they're thinking and are they secretly blaming you. You don't know, do you?

Jill Johnson

"Now he's playing happy families"

Jill Johnson is 43 and a restaurant manager. She tells her story calmly. Asked a question, she answers it and then stops, not inclined to elaborate, waiting for the next question. She rarely elaborates without being prompted. She seems concerned that her daughter, Claire, who is now 19 and was abused by Jill's ex-partner, Morris, has never accepted the need for counselling or joining the course at the Partners for Protection programme, from which she herself has benefited. She lived with Morris, her husband's cousin, someone she had known most of her life. She has three children, two with her husband and one with her second partner. She and her offending partner had no children together. He has two daughters by a previous relationship and now has two stepdaughters of infant-school age by the woman he went to live with after the abuse occurred and his relationship with Jill ended. It later emerged that he had been arrested for gross indecency when he was 16. Claire was abused by Morris when she was 11. Jill is now in a new relationship and has a grandchild. The impression she gives is that, despite a quiet anger that her partner has never paid for what he did, she is telling of events which are (mostly) now behind her.

We had a good relationship and I had known him since I was 16. He was four years older than me. He was me husband's cousin. He abused me daughter when she was 11 and she's 19 now. She told her teacher at school and I got a phone call at work to say could I go into school and social services and the police were there. I was shocked 'cos it actually had happened two years previously – she had waited two years before she told anybody. I was shocked that it happened, 'cos it's something I never expected from him. I believed me daughter.

He actually worked at the school: he was an IT technician. He got suspended that day and social services told him he would have to leave the house until we found out how things were going, not have any contact, so he left.

I didn't speak to him that day but on the phone later when he'd gone to stay with me eldest son, 'cos he had nowhere else to go. He didn't deny it; he said he couldn't remember the incident 'cos he was drunk. I didn't think a lot about it, to be honest, I was so angry with him, I was shocked by it all, trying to understand why it took her so long to say anything and at the same time I was looking after a toddler. That was another thing that was hard to understand because he had two daughters, one's older than mine and one's younger and, I mean, they were always together at weekends when they came to stay. The fact he was a dad and he had girls, so it's something you didn't expect. He also worked in a comprehensive school, and you don't get jobs like that if there is anything people should know about.

Me daughter said at the time that she didn't want anything to go any further forward so the police took a step back. Because I was happy, she didn't want to make us unhappy. She wanted to say to him, "I forgive you." I felt very bad because, as I said, to her me happiness was more important. She was talking about me happiness because later on she made it known that she was happiest when it was me and her and she felt a bit out when me partner came along. She was 7 when her brother was born and she liked that, but she liked that we'd been together on our own.

We had social services' involvement for nearly two year. Sometimes, I felt at the meetings, "Why am I sitting here?", and sometimes you'd think, "Well, if I had been a better mother I wouldn't have been here." There was no anger toward people at the meetings but I think I withdrew quite a bit. I went more into myself when we were having all these meetings 'cos there would be two people from social services there and the person who used to do the access, giving their opinion of things, and the school giving their opinion of things, and I used to think everybody's talking about me and talking about me children half the time as if I'm not there.

Then, about 18 months to two years, me daughter wanted to make charges because I don't think she could put a close to it herself. She decided to go to the police. They came round and took statements, and it went in front of the criminal board or whatever it is [the Crown Prosecution Service] and they said they weren't going pursue it. They said because he had treatment – social services put him on a course: it was the Sexual Behaviour Unit [in Newcastle] he went to – and because it was such a while, it wasn't worth them prosecuting, basically. She thinks it's as if he's gotten away with it all. I felt the same thing, really, that he's turned our lives upside down and he's going on as if there's nothing the matter with his life.

He was actually involved all the time we were going to social services meetings because me daughter went through a stage where she wanted to be a family again, she wanted everybody to just go away and leave her alone. So he was involved that way, and he used to have supervised access to them [the children] and then that stopped when she decided to stop it all. He saw the little one as his own, 'cos he's little and he's never seen his real dad.

It stopped when me daughter went to one of the meetings and said that she no longer wanted to be a family unit, she wanted it to just be me and her and her brother, and she didn't want any more involvement with him; we stopped access there and then. Now we have no contact at all. I have seen him because he's been in the school yard 'cos he now has a new family. He doesn't know where to look. I would like to go over and hit him, especially since it's two little girls he's picking up from school.

She's the one that saw him first in the school yard. I was with her; I didn't see, it's a good size yard. She just turned round and says "Have you noticed that he's over there with [name] waiting in the school yard. How dare he?"

He lives in the same house as we lived in. I moved out so he could move back in. It's less than three miles.

I don't know if his new partner knows. I went to see the headmistress 'cos obviously the school was involved all the way through it, and she said she had been made aware that he was in the school yard. She had contacted the authorities and he hasn't been in for the last six weeks so I don't know if they've been and stepped in 'cos obviously they wouldn't give me any information.

Sometimes I don't try to think of it at all because me daughter wants to just get on with her life now, but we had a very bad couple of years. I feel guilty a lot of the time because I'm her mam, I'm supposed to protect her.

She went through a stage where she was ... well, it was hard to say sometimes because if it was because of this or because she was a teenager, but she did run away from home a few times; she would be very violent at times. She would break things; she hit the dog with so much force once she actually broke a knuckle – really! She went through a stage when she became a goth, where she covered herself from head to foot so nobody could say what she looked like when she started developing. So much so that we rowed and I actually hit her once which was the first time ever in her entire life and she got me arrested.

With me, it was a case of no point in hating him, 'cos he wasn't feeling what I was feeling. The only person I was hurting in the long run would be meself and I think because I started to feel like that and I was a lot more calmer, she started to get a lot more calmer. I mean, now we don't argue, she'll discuss things now and she doesn't hold things back any more and I think now she's sort of like, "He's not going get the better of us, I'm going live me life now."

Because of the incident, I don't have as much trust in people as I would have. It's awful really 'cos sometimes you think the sinister side of people when they could be quite innocent. I'd been with somebody that I have known me whole entire adult life. There was a lot of trust there and then finding out he could do a thing like that was even more hard to understand. If it had been somebody I had known a year or so and didn't really know about them, but I knew about his failed relationship, I knew about his children. When I was married to me husband, they had the same family bonds. Do you know what I mean? That somebody you had known that long, to find out they could do something like that, yes, you are more wary of people that you don't really know.

I'm more protective of me children because of it. I am more wary of the little one. He's always been taught not to talk to strangers, but even more so now, I'm more protective of him. You know, he likes to go to the shop by himself and I say, "No, I'll stand here, I can watch you all the time," and he'll say, "I'm all right, I'm all right," and I know he's all right but I still like to … I'm a bit over-protective.

It's strange, in a certain way it makes us understand something with me dad. He brought me and me three brothers up by himself. I didn't have a mam at all and me dad was always very wary about cuddling us and things like that, and I used to think me dad didn't love us and was a bit standoffish but now I can see now why he was like that. He was always frightened that people would take that affection towards me wrongly because it was an all-male environment I was brought up in.

Me brothers – I've got five now, but I only had three when I was at home – they don't know about this [the abuse of Claire]. I just told them that the relationship broke up. He's [Morris] an only child but I spoke to his mam and dad, but it was his cousins I was close to – they used to baby-sit me eldest laddie when he was little – so I knew he was close to a few of his cousins. His mam and dad don't know because I had nothing to do with them after I left, after it came out; I had nothing to do with them at all. The only person that was involved was his daughters' mam. She stopped the daughters having anything to do with him.

The teachers were very good actually. Claire's teacher liked her quite a lot and she was even nice enough that when we stopped going for some meetings because I didn't have any transport at the time, she would actually say, "Come to the school and I'll take you with me," and she would bring us back. They tried their best all the time with us.

The police were fine but I thought social services kept us in the dark about things. I felt like I was just a number sometimes rather than an individual person. They would say that they were doing things and I didn't feel that they were actually because things would take so long to get to the end, you know. I mean I had them in me life nearly two year. I know they had a job to do, but I felt like they weren't really helping me with how I was coping with things, I got more help coming here [to the Partners for Protection course] than I ever did off social services.

The people that were coming here were in similar circumstances as me, we were all here with children that had been abused so the other mums sort of knew, like, what we were all going through. I mean, the social worker she hadn't been in that situation, she was just somebody doing her job. When you talk to people and you find out they've got the same feelings, you don't feel like you're the only one and they understand how you feel. To a certain extent, I had nobody to turn to; I couldn't turn to me family because with them being all brothers their reaction would have been basically to go and kill him. I didn't know how to cope with how me daughter was feeling and since I didn't know anybody that had been through the same thing. How could I find out how to cope with what she was going through?

I wasn't forced to come here [to the Partners for Protection course] but I was told it was in the best interests of the case that I did and they [social services] told me it was like a good parenting guide thing and that made me feel as if I was a bad parent. They made us feel that if I didn't come here it would look bad against me 'cos they were doing reports on how Jo was doing at school; they were also doing reports of how me youngest was doing at school and yet he wasn't involved in it. I was being judged all the time, being judged on being a parent and being judged on not knowing it [the abuse] was happening. Basically, they were saying there was signs there, why didn't I see them? If I had known, who would I have told? Who'd be the right people to tell? Do you go to the police, social services, your GP – who do you see?

I don't really know what the signs were supposed to be, but to me the way she acted at times was as a teenager. I mean, she was at a funny age, but she always got on very well with him so if she had been not wanting to be in the same room as him, or not wanting to be with him … and because he worked at her school, she used to go to school with him every morning and come home with him every night – to me that's not a child that's doesn't want to be around that person.

I didn't feel [at the Partners for Protection course] any more as if I was the only parent going through this. I would say I came out a more positive, stronger person than I did when I first started coming. I didn't feel any more that it was me fault, you know, I didn't do that to her, it was him and it wasn't my fault that I didn't realise he was abusing her. They made us understand how they [offenders] can manipulate you as well as manipulate the child; for you not to know what's going on, that it wasn't me being a bad parent.

Claire told me eldest son. When she ran away from home that time he seen her – he had a place of his own – and he went and got her and he asked her why and she told him. He just come to me and he says, "She's told us why she's run away", so he said what she told him and he was very angry, not with me, with him for what he did, and he felt bad as well because he's, you know, the older child. He said he should have been protecting his sister and I says, "Well, you weren't living at home." He was very angry with him that he could do it. He doesn't shout, but you can tell in his tone; he goes deep, deeper and you know he's angry, but he's not a shouter.

He didn't know what to do, because, as I said, he [Morris] got told that he had to leave the house when they were starting the investigation, and he actually went to stay with me son in his house. Me son did ask what's going on, but he [Morris] said that he wasn't sure, said that it had something to do with me and the children and that's all he said to him. Me son's not the type to ask; unless you tell him, he won't ask.

I'm angry that he's never paid any price for what he did because me and me daughter are the ones that's suffered and he's gotten away with it as if it was nothing and I know he was put on this [sex offenders'] course, but he didn't even finish the course, so he didn't even finish his punishment as such and now he's playing happy families. I just feel he hasn't got the right to be a father figure in any child's life.

Me daughter's a very straight-talking young lady, sometimes too straight I would say, but she gets on well with everybody. She won't tolerate anybody she doesn't like; she has very much a mind of her own. I would say she came out of what happened different. She has always been a child that knew her own mind and would do it in any case, but I think she went through a stage where she just wanted everybody to be happy and I think that's why she didn't say anything for so long because she wanted me to be happy, and then she went through the rebellion stage where she hated everybody, whereas now it's a case of she knows she's an adult. It wasn't my fault, it was his fault, and she just wants to look forward. She's at college, she knows she wants to go to uni [versity] and she knows what she wants to do with her life.

Clare Truman

"I want to go back with him 'cos I love him"

Clare Truman is a very open, jolly 22-year-old who laughs a lot. She lives on benefits and is the mother of Becky, who is 8. Her daughter was born when she was in a violent former relationship. She met Nathan Fell, who is 32 and had himself been in care after being brought up with a violent father. They lived together for nearly two years before three allegations of past sexual offending by Nathan came to light, one as recently as three years ago, but there is no suggestion that he has ever abused Becky. He had not told Clare anything about his past. He has a son, Darryl, who is in care, by a previous relationship with Michelle. Despite the devastation that this has brought to her – frequent abuse from neighbours, social isolation, separation from most of her family and friends – Clare is fighting for Nathan to be allowed to live with her and her daughter again. She speaks in a tone that suggests her frustration that they cannot be together and the certainty she feels that she can protect her child if they are able to do so. Clare is one of those rare interviewees who refers to her partner by his first name: several other interviewees refer to their husbands and partners as "he".

I met Nathan in March 2005 on the drink in the town and it just developed from there really. I had me daughter, Becky, and that was when I was in a violent relationship with her dad, but I'd split with him in June/July 2004, so I'd been on me own for quite a while. There was court hearings 'cos he broke into me house and things. I dunno, me and Nathan just got a friendship and it moved on from there, really. He was there for us through the court case [about her child' access] and things, and it just developed from there really.

It was just a normal relationship, I suppose. We had our ups and downs, you know, normal arguments, nothing really drastic. It was really good, really good. There was a lot of issues around like when we used to go out with his friends for a drink and they would come back he was upset 'cos he hasn't got access to his son, but I used to say to him, "Well go and see a solicitor about it," and he would just say, "All right, I will," but it never ever happened.

Last New Year's Eve [2006], he'd gone out on the drink, and he'd come back and he was full of hell, just wanted an argument. So I says to him, "Just go to your mother's, blah, blah, blah," so he left in the next morning. He phoned us but I wasn't prepared to talk to him so I just hung up the phone and I phoned him back later that morning and he was at his son's mother's house and I says, "When you're finished there come home and have a talk and things." He came home and he was dead upset. He was told that his son was in care, he'd never known anything about this and he was gonna fight for him and even then I didn't know anything. He was getting in touch with social services and things.

It was 5 February this year and I had a knock on the door and it was child protection and they took Nathan and me into the kitchen 'cos me neighbour was in the living room as she was asking Nathan to do painting and decorating. They says, "What do you know about Nathan and Nathan's background?" I was a bit confused at the time and I says, "I know there's issues with him and his son; he hasn't got contact with his son," and they just said to Nathan, "Do you wanna tell her the rest?" and he went, "No, not really." I was then taken into the living room and I was foaming. Obviously, they'd introduced their-selves as child protection so all this was tumbling through me mind. Nathan made a statement. There was the police officer who was there from child protection and I was with the social worker from child protection.

The social worker asked me neighbour if she would be prepared to take Becky just out for an hour or so 'cos things needed to be sorted out. Me neighbour was on her way up the stairs with Becky to go and to get her ready to take her out and the social worker asked me, had me daughter ever been left alone with Nathan, so straight away there was alarm bells for me but also for me neighbour. So, she got Becky ready and off they went and Nathan was asked to leave. A statement was read out – I cannot really remember the date – but when he was 13 … it was an indecent assault, he indecently assaulted, I think it was, a 5 or a 6-year-old boy. Then when he was 14 he was accused of indecently assaulting a 5-year-old girl (that was his niece), and then, in 2003, he was accused of indecently assaulting his son.

He was cautioned about the 5-year-old girl because there was evidence that she had been abused, but there was no evidence of who abused her and, I don't know, it was explained that because of the laws at the time and things, it just … it never went ahead.

I was only given them brief details. He was took in for questioning regard-ing his son, but no charges were brought but I had to get all the details. They said to me they couldn't tell me the ins and outs of what had happened, that was down to Nathan. So off I trotted to where he was [staying] with his mam to try and drum the truth out of him and it took him two days to tell us every-thing. He still denies the past two but admits to the first one when he was 13.

It was a huge shock, 'cos he had been living with us for just short of two year. I mean Becky's me daughter and she called him dad; he'd looked after her loads of times because I never, ever suspected anything of him. It was a huge shock – huge!

I did have worries about Becky at first 'cos I thought he's been left with her loads of times, he's bathed her loads of times … I mean when we first got toge-ther she was in nappies, so he used to change her nappy and I just thought,

"Oh my God!" And I still think, you know, he's done all these things and not told me, so he's put me and Becky in a … in a very funny position but I can put me hand on me heart and say I don't think he has ever done anything to Becky 'cos I've, like, lived the past two year in me head over and over, day by day and just nothing's rang any alarm bells; he's never been over keen to be alone with her.

She was in a council nursery and they had positive reports, nothing untoward with her behaviour 'cos she used to attend three full days a week. Everyone was quite happy with her development and what have you. She was never scared, she still asks for him 'cos there is no contact allowed at the minute. We're still fighting to be a family again and she still asks for him to this day, she wants her daddy to come home, so it's quite stressful really.

[Why do you want to go back with him?] 'Cos I love him. Obviously, I've attended [the Partners for Protection course] and I just feel that everything they've told us about the different behaviours and things like … that Nathan's never … 'cos I've lived with him for two year … he's never displayed any of these behaviours. I know there will have to be a child protection plan in place and I'm willing to stick to that, I've discussed it with Nathan at length and I've told him that if we're allowed to be a family again he wouldn't be allowed to bath her, he wouldn't be allowed to get her ready and things like that, and he's just said, "Well, whatever needs to be done."

Nobody, like me parents, knew about this when it happened but they know about it now. Me mam and dad just went off him because … well, obviously … With the neighbour being there, when I was being told this, she was telling people straight away, that he was abusing this kid, that kid, just not even knowing the truth, not even knowing the full story. "Oh, social services have knocked on Clare's door, they're asking has Nathan ever been left alone with me bairn, you know what that means, blah, blah, blah," and it went on like that for a while and it was just a nightmare. Everyone on the street knew about it.

I had loads of abuse shouted at us and things like that and then I think it was May [2007], me mam and dad were out drinking, they had just come off a week's holiday and they were told in the pub. One of me … well, a lass that used to be me friend turned around to me mam and went, "Oh how's your Clare?" Me mam went, "Oh she's still trying to move, blah, blah, blah," 'cos I'd just always told me mam I wanted to move because I'm having trouble with the neighbours, but I didn't actually tell them the real reason. And she went, "Yeah, I know it's terrible about Nathan being a paedophile," so the shit just hit the fan really and they came round all guns blazing and me dad says, "As long as I live, I'm having nothing to do with him," and he wants nothing to do with me. Me mam was a bit more understanding, she just sat there and listened to it all, and so it's really me dad still, he's still not happy, he doesn't really talk to us.

I was in the town with me mam a couple of weeks ago and, you know, she was saying, "You know I'm not happy about the situation etc., etc.," and I just says, "mam but I love him, he's hurt me, he's hurt us really bad but I love him. I tried hating him." Doing [the course], you know, there was people there that's saying that their kids have been abused and hard it's been for them, or they have been abused how hard it's been for them, and all the time I was thinking Nathan has done this to a family – whether the second two happened or not – he has done this to a family and I tried me hardest to hate him, but I just can't.

Me mam had said, like if it come to light that it was just juvenile, you know, confusion, she would understand 'cos then she disclosed to me that something had happened to her when she was younger. She was 8 and the boy was 14 and something happened to her, which I was really shocked at 'cos me mam never told me that before. She said she still sees the bloke now, so she totally understands how people can change, how there could have just been confusion, but she's ... me mam's still up in arms about her feelings because nobody knows the truth.

They're [neighbours] doing it 'cos Nathan's not there, I suppose. I've had text messages on me phone. It even happens now when I walk past a certain house, taking me daughter to school, she shouts abuse – that neighbour that was in me house that day – just anything she can think of really. She just comes to her window, opens her window and shouts.

She was me friend, quite pally. She had a granddaughter that visited her often and she would often come down and have cups of tea. They were getting laminate flooring put down once and they'd asked Nathan to go and shift furniture and things like that. Everyone on the street used to ask Nathan to go in and do the odd jobs and things like that. Would Nathan mind doing a bit of painting and decorating? Would he mind changing this fuse? Would he mind ... you know what I mean, whatever.

Nathan just always wanted to tell me but as time went on it got harder and as things got better between us, it was harder and I am not defending him, but I can, in a way, understand where he was coming from because I don't suppose it is a very nice thing to tell somebody, but I'm still very annoyed that he didn't.

Me sister, she's quite supportive. She's me youngest sister, she's 21. She is living with her fiancé and things. She was the only one I could talk to really when I found out. I think it was mebbe a couple of weeks after I found out and let the shock settle down but I went to them straight away, 'cos I just had to have somebody to talk to. I went and told her and just her, her and her partner, that I couldn't believe it. They were quite shocked, but they said they would support me in whatever decision I wanted to make. I told me parents that they would react the way they did; fear really.

[*How did you feel you had been dealt with by the authorities like social services?*] Crap! Totally, totally ... it's just been horrible, it really has. When it all first came out, you know I was between two posts really: do I walk away from it or do a fight for it or do I still wanna be with him? Do I wanna leave him? They bullied us to give them a decision. I wasn't given a vast amount of time to make me mind up. When our Becky was being cared for by me mam and dad or by me sister and I was speaking to Nathan and getting more bits and pieces of information and things and he was just saying that me and Becky mean the world to him and things like that really. He was absolutely devastated and so was I, the pair of us … were just in bits. I just decided that I loved him and I would stick by him and do everything the authorities asked us to do but then I was left for about two or three months, just on me own with nothing.

There was no intervention from social services, although I was promised a social worker. Like I say, I just had nothing. I was getting abuse from me neighbours and the police were saying, "You have got to tell your social worker," and I'm saying, "I haven't got one." And then one day I'd just had enough. I was staying at me mam's quite a lot, still her not knowing then – she just thought me and Nathan were going through a rough patch and that we were on a break and that Becky wasn't going to see him because we didn't know how things were gonna pan out for us. One day I'd just had enough and I phoned the original social worker that was involved, and I told her. I says, "Look", I says, "I cannot go on like this no more, I'm getting abuse from me neighbours, I don't know where I am, I don't know what I'm meant to be doing." I says, "All I've been told is that Becky can't have any contact with Nathan, but other than that I'm on me own." I was in tears and things. We put a complaint in, and by 4 o'clock that afternoon I had a social worker, so I feel like I only got a social worker because I complained.

Then the next day I went to meet me social worker at the office and she says, "Oh, I'm new, I don't know your case. To be honest I don't really know what I'm doing," and I thought, "Fantastic! I haven't just been given a social worker 'cos I've complained, I've been given a social worker that hasn't got a clue what she's doing." She makes appointments and then cancels them at the last minute, but it seems to be all the time, she's always off, she never gives us a straight answer, she's not very supportive. Every time she comes out she just says, "I haven't got a quick fix," but this has been going on for like ten months now and we're still no further forward.

When we've been going to [case] conferences, the local authority said the only chance me and Nathan had of being together is me attending Mosaic. I came to Mosaic and really enjoyed the course and really found it alarming but I just enjoyed it. But me social worker … they used to come out every week and say, "How's it going?" and I'd say that I really enjoyed it. They went, "You enjoyed it? It's not something you should enjoy." But I just enjoyed it for the company 'cos I was so isolated, I still am really, I still don't really talk to anybody about it, none of me neighbours speak to us, but I just enjoyed it 'cos we were all in the same boat. We used to have a really good laugh on the course, we didn't judge each other. Towards the end we were like mates really, rather than just a group that met once a week.

The police were a bit more supportive. I was told that if anything happened that me number was flagged so if ever I had any abuse, anything at all that I was worried about to dial 999 and the police would be straight there. There was one morning I was out and me immediate neighbour – she's still quite pally with us – I'd knocked on her door for something and the woman on the end, who I still get bother with to this day, she was seeing somebody out of her house and she says, "That's her, the nonce blah, blah, blah," and all this abuse came out. It was about quarter to twelve when mothers were coming past with their kids from nursery and things; it was just horrendous. So, I goes in a bit of a state, ran in the house dialled 999 and I got knocked out of bed at two in the morning by the police. They said they were there about the complaint I'd made and they went, "Oh well, we have just drove past there and they're all in bed so we'll just leave it." So it went onto be a bit of a farce like that but then it got passed on to our local beat bobby and he was quite supportive. He took a statement off us on all the incidents that had happened, he went and warned her unofficially, just to wind her neck in sort of thing. It continued so he went back up and she had to sign his pocket book, but the problem they've got is that it died down for a period of time and now it's started again so everything's up in the air on what they can do really.

Social services have said to me a couple of times, "You know, we can't understand why you want to be with him, you're dead intelligent," and things like that. But they've said, "We wouldn't be in your life if it wasn't for him," but they've never ever said that I should have known or anything like that.

I find it really hard to get round in me head because I've said to him [Nathan] loads of times, "Why, why?" and you just ... he's said a couple of times, "Oh, I was off me nut," 'cos he had drug problems when he was younger, he used to get beat up by his father, him and his dad didn't have a very good relationship. His mam says he was always naughty as a child. He just said he was baby sitting one night and got off his nut and stripped this laddie down and touched him and I was like, "You cannot use that as an excuse," so something must have been there and he just said, "I was a bit confused and that was it." He's been through assessments, not lately, but he has been through an assessment at the SBU [Sexual Behaviour Unit] in Newcastle. They said that offence wasn't premeditated, therefore he acted on impulse so, yes, he poses a risk, but it's not ... it could be a controlled risk not major, major risk and he's had ... he did have work undertaken.

But the problem we've got at the minute is that social services still see ... you see, 'cos there's two local authorities involved, Newcastle with his son and North Tyneside with me and Becky. Newcastle are doing a psychological assessment, they've got no intentions in their proceedings to do another SBU assessment, but North Tyneside are concerned about the sexual risk, but are refusing to do an SBU assessment because it costs money. Social services said the SBU says there's no way they would be happy to assess him because unless he admits to something else the outcome's gonna be the same.

To be perfectly honest, I'm not sure about the second one with his niece, because obviously there was evidence that she had been abused but they couldn't pin it on Nathan. The niece was saying that it was Nathan but there was no evidence that it was actually Nathan, there was just evidence there that she had been abused. But where his son's concerned I don't think he did.

The son's mother made the allegation and the son wasn't examined. He was taken for an interview and it was all recorded, but nothing was disclosed. His son was only 4 at the time and he has never disclosed anything in front of the social worker or the police officer about Nathan and Michelle [Nathan's former partner]. Michelle said that Darryl had gone to her saying all these things but Darryl's never ever come forward and said whether he has or he hasn't.

Nathan, he has been given leave of the no contact order [he is not allowed to see his son] so obviously there has been a lot of questions put to Darryl and he's just said he doesn't know if his dad's ever abused him or not, and, like, he's 8 now which is quite confusing for everybody because ... I dunno ...

If it was proved about his niece, I'm not sure how I would feel to be honest. I believe there's a possibility he did because obviously with his conviction, there was a lot of social workers involved because his dad was very, very violent to Nathan at that time. Nathan was actually taken into care and put into a home. There was quite a lot of supervision orders and the only place he could go was his sister Lisa's to stay for the weekend, but this is where the niece was – she was Lisa's daughter. Nathan was still taking a lot of drugs and things so I believe there's a possibility that it did happen, but even now seeing Nathan and this niece, there's just nothing there, nothing that she's scared of about him, nothing ... she doesn't treat him any different to any other of her aunties or uncles or anything. If it was beyond doubt that he abused Darryl I would walk away because he's had treatment done, obviously it would be far too high a risk and I just ... I dunno, I couldn't forgive him because it's too recent, it was only four ... three year ago.

All this has made me, like, I can't trust anybody. I was always a very trustworthy person, a very trusting person, you know, and now I just think because of the way people have reacted to me ... you know, they've all shouted abuse at us but they've never actually come up to me and said. "Looka, we've heard this duh, duh, duh ... what's going on?" – nobody's ever done that. Like I say, the only person on me street that speaks to us is me immediate next-door neighbour, everybody else has just walked away, gone off their own way. They were meant to be me friends. I can understand to some degree but, I dunno, I just don't seem to trust anybody, I haven't got the time of day for anybody, I don't go out me way to speak to people 'cos I used to always be nice to everybody – do you know what I mean? – and now I just feel like I cannot be bothered with it because it's all false.

Even the people that don't know, which isn't very many, they'll stop to speak to us and they'll say, "I fell out with such and such duh, duh," and I just think I cannot be bothered with this, the general day-to-day arguments, the general tittle-tattle and things like that. So I've isolated meself quite a bit really because I feel angry, I just feel hurt, but not just by Nathan but by me friends as well, or people who were meant to be me friends. I'm a quite forward person and I think if this came out about somebody else in the street and me daughter had been spending time with them, rather than shouting abuse at them and things I would just go to them and say, "Looka, what's happened, because me daughter's been part of this whatever?" But I'm very much like that, I'm very much straightforward and I don't really judge people a lot anyway; I'm quite laid back. I'm just more angry at the fact that everybody's quick to jump to conclusions about … they all think Nathan's abused me … abused Becky, they all think Nathan's abused X, Y and Z, but they don't know, and they've never ever come and asked, do you know what I mean? It just annoys us, really, really annoys us.

Like I say, I totally understand their reaction to a certain degree, but I just wish somebody would come up and say, "What's really happened?" instead of shouting all this abuse. I mean, to be honest, before all this happened to me, I never really thought about it; I mean there is all kinds of different sex offenders, whether it be rapists or … I thought they [sex offenders] should all be … they were paedophiles, things like that. It just scares you, doesn't it, and you think, "Oh, my God". But I think doing this course, there is a difference between a paedophile and a sex offender. Nathan's classed as a sex offender, but he's not on the sex offenders' register because his conviction was so long ago.

Nathan hates it, what's happened. When it was all quite really bad at first, oh, he just … when I used to phone him, he used to cry about it, he used to apologise and he still does, and I say, "You should have told us," and … I dunno, he's just so … he just keeps on saying, "I'm so sorry for putting you through what I've put you through," and he's dead grateful that I'm sticking by him but there's nothing he can do, nothing he can do. He'll say if anything happens, "Have you phoned the police? Have you phoned the social worker? Have you done this, have you done that?" but there's nothing you can do now; it's done, isn't it? That's not the view he takes; it's not, "Well it's done now, so get on with it". It's the view I take 'cos I just think it's more a hindrance to us now than an upset, do you know what I mean? And I just think, "Well, they've got nothing better to do, so just get on with it."

We had a [case] conference in October [2007] and our local authority had said they would wait for the outcome of the psychological assessment. Me solicitor argued the point, you know, you're not worried about the psychological side, you're worried about the sexual side so they're saying they'll reconsider in March [2008], see what the outcome is. But me solicitor says the outcome in March could be they're still not gonna assess him. Where does it leave you? So at the minute me solicitor's wrote to the local authority and said that I'm no longer willing to stick to the child protection plan – that I've given them plenty days notice – that I'm gonna let Nathan have contact with Becky again and I'm going to be responsible. Me solicitor's advised us that they could start care proceedings but in the care proceedings we can ask for an SBU assessment. I'll force their hand. Me solicitor says it's just a technicality to get them to do what we want them to do.

Ann Baker

"I'll be honest with you – I just want to have a happy life now"

At 23, Ann Baker, a former cleaner who now works as a care assistant, was married to John Baker, a man 26 years her senior. They had three daughters. A decade ago, when one daughter, Louise, was 17, he died while having sex with a friend of hers. On the day of his funeral, Louise disclosed to her mother that he had been abusing her since she was 7 years old. After her father died, Louise began a relationship with his son, Colin Barton, Ann's stepson, and they had a son, 4-year-old Lewis. Colin Barton later abducted and sexually assaulted a child who was a stranger to him. Aged 37, he is now serving a life sentence for that offence. Neither of Ann's two brothers nor her sister speak to her and her relationship with her 70-year-old father, never close, is now even more distant. Louise, now 26, and her son live with Ann and Ann's new partner, Robert.

I was married about 21 years and, like all people, you think it is such a perfect marriage. He couldn't do enough for us; he'd spoil us – whatever I wanted I got. I worked full time because me partner was poorly: he did work in the beginning – he was a painter and decorator – but he had to give up work because he had heart problems. He had lots of problems so he was mostly the main carer for me children because I was working full time, so he'd done everything for them, bathed them, fed them and everything, apart from if I was off weekends and then we'd go out as a family. Brilliant, lovely, nothing, no suspicions or nothing, and it went on like that, as I say, up until he died. Me and the two youngest daughters were in Manchester on that day, because I had took them down to see the Spice Girls. Louise didn't go with us, Louise stopped back.

When we came out I phoned the house to let him know that we were out of the theatre and we were travelling back up with friends but I couldn't get no answer from the phone, which was unusual, so I rang me parents' house to see if they knew where he was because I knew he was poorly that morning. Me father came on the phone and he said, "I've got some bad news for you." I says, "What's happened?" He said, "John's died." Well, I just collapsed with shock and the two younger daughters, they were hysterical.

We got back home and I went straight to me mam's house because Louise was there because they had been up and brought her down and Louise was just cowering in the corner and I thought why is she cowering in the corner? I know she was in shock. She was 16–17 at the time and we went home, but she didn't want to come back to the house because he died in the house. I said, "We need to go back home, Louise," so we all went back. We got some sleep that night and then the next day they got the doctor out and the police were out because it was a sudden death and then I found out that what had happened.

Louise had just got her own flat with a friend, and her dad asked her to bring her friend up to the house so he could have, you know, sexual intercourse with her but the girl did not want to come up at first and he offered her money and she said "Yes," so they came up to the house her and her dad says to Louise, "You go out and don't come back too early, don't come back too quick." So she went out, she was very upset because she knew what was going to happen. When she came back her friend was hysterical at the top of the stairs. She said, "Louise, Louise, come quick there is something wrong with your dad." So Louise went up. She came running back down the stairs and went to see a next-door neighbour, got her to come because she was scared, and when the neighbour went upstairs there he was, dead.

We had done the funeral, and that day, on the tea-time, Louise came to us and says, "mam, I need to speak to you." I says, "What's wrong?" and she goes, "I don't know how you are going to take this but I need to tell you now." I says, "What's wrong, Louise?" because it wasn't like Louise, you know: she told me everything, we were really close. She said, "mam", she says, "I've got to tell you – me dad has been sexually abusing me." She says, "I think I was about 7." She couldn't remember exactly from what age but she knew she was young. I just couldn't believe it, I believed her because I knew Louise wouldn't lie to us. I says, "Why couldn't you tell us before?" and she said, "mam, I couldn't." She says, "He threatened us." He used to threaten her with knives, he said that if she told me they [her sisters] would get taken away, he would hurt her sisters, they would never see us again. She said, "I couldn't do it, I was so scared."

This had been going on from when she was 7 until he died but he was still involving her friends in the activities and used to make Louise sit and watch whatever was happening.

I'll be honest with you, no – nothing, nothing came across to us like that. It was a normal family life; there was nothing there to give me reason to worry about anything, you know, nothing at all. It quite shocked us, the only thing is that – and now, since I did the Partners for Protection [programme], that has really clicked in place – thinking back he was grooming me, and I didn't realise he was grooming me so he could keep on abusing Louise the way he was. I mean, he would do anything I wanted; what I wanted, I would get. He would say to us, "You can go out with your friends for a night out," and I thought, well he has got the children all the time, I'm at work, surely he would want a break but he still managed, and thinking back now this was all part of his plan to get what he wanted.

What happened shattered us, it really shattered us, because I thought it was perfect and I really loved him, I really loved him, but as soon as that came out,

I just … I hated him and everything. I'm still angry now because I couldn't confront him, he'd died and I couldn't confront him, I couldn't do nothing, so for 10 years I have had this and I haven't been able to do nothing about it until I come to this [Partners for Protection programme] and it only came out because of what Colin done otherwise I had no one. I didn't know what to do. I couldn't do nothing and that was so annoying. I didn't know where to go, I didn't know what to do. It just really wore me down, I was depressed, just really low, I just let meself go really.

It was hard for them [the other children] to accept. They were very upset about it, they couldn't believe it and it's still hard for them now, to be honest. They do accept it now but it's took a long time. But, do you know what I don't really know? I don't know what they thought about Louise. They seemed to … I don't know, they loved their dad, he never hurt them, so why would he hurt Louise? I think they must have been a bit – how can I put it? – there must have been a bit of hate there towards Louise because of what she said, but they get on fine now. It was a bit difficult, too, because I wanted to comfort Louise, but I felt awful because I couldn't do nothing to like, help her. As I say, I didn't know where to go to, I didn't know where to go for help, you know, and what could they have done? He wasn't there for them to do anything, he couldn't go to prison, he couldn't go to court.

Louise always said she never, ever blamed me, because she knew I didn't know what was happening and she didn't want me to know; she has never ever blamed me. We were very close, very close and the two other girls, we are close as well, always have been with me. The three girls have always been close. I believed Louise straight away, yes, I did, and what I said to them [the other two children] was, "You must believe Louise because Louise is not going to say something like this if it hasn't happened." It seemed all right after that. They were very close to their dad and he never actually touched them, never hurt them. It was all down to Louise that they never got touched, because Louise said she would do anything he asked her to do to protect her sisters, so she took a lot on, you know.

I had to be open about what had happened with the family because I was very close to me mam, not so close to me dad, but me mam. I had never ever met me partner's family, no one on his side at all. Me family were shocked, very shocked, but, you see, the problem was me parents didn't want me to marry him in the beginning because of the age difference – there was a 26-year age difference between us – and I think that made me more determined to marry him because they were against it, so they weren't happy about us being with him anyway. I regret it now, I really do. I wish I had listened to them, but do kids listen to their parents? Oh! I had a brilliant childhood, a really good childhood, I really enjoyed me childhood, no problems at all. I was born in Preston Hospital, North Shields, which is pulled down now. Me mam was born in North Shields and so was me dad. I just remember all the holidays we used to go on, big family holidays though, we used to go to a place called Ovington, it was like little bungalows and that; we used to rent them. There used to be a big stream: I can still see it now. There was me, me sister, two brothers and then there was me uncles and aunties and their kids and, you know, I really enjoyed it, really nice, nice summer holidays they were. I had no bothers, no troubles.

They were really loving, me parents, they really were. Me dad used to like going for a drink as well, so sometimes when he come in, mam would say be quiet because they're – meaning us children – in bed and they would have an argument like anybody would and that was the only problem. Me mam didn't like him drinking but, no, no, no, there was never any physical violence; nothing like that. I take after him, I'm a worrier and me dad's always been a worrier. I worry about the least little thing, me, I do, I worry all the time, I get very stressed, very stressed if nothing's going right in the house. They hate it when I'm in a stressed mood. They say, "Oh me mam's on one again, keep out of her way," but I cannot help it, I've always been like that. If nothing's going right for us, I get meself in such a titty you know it's, er … but I've always been the same and me dad's like that.

Of course, when me mam and dad heard what had happened, that just didn't help matters, but they did back us up. Me mam was great, she was brilliant. Unfortunately she died; in fact she died before this happened about Colin, which I am glad because she didn't like Colin at all. You see because he was me stepson – he was John's son. Although John always said that Colin's mam had had an affair with somebody in London because John was meant to be in prison for some reason at the time. Are you with us now? It's very complicated, very complicated. Him and Louise – do you want us to tell you about this part? – well, him and Louise took a house on together because Colin had nowhere to go, so Louise says, "You can stop with me." They got into a relationship because her dad always said that Colin wasn't his son – he was but he always said he wasn't, so him and Louise got closer.

Me dad was very bitter, very bitter about what John had done to his granddaughter and bitter because he said, "I warned you not to marry him." In fact, not over what John did but the Colin situation, I've lost all me family now, they don't speak to us. Me dad will speak to us if I go down to see him, but, apart from that, me brothers and sisters just disowned us. A few year ago, I was at the shops and me sister come to us and all of a sudden she just blurted it out, she says, "I can't understand you!" I says, "What do you mean?" She says, "I can't believe you didn't know it was happening to your own daughter." I tried to tell her I didn't know, but she can't understand how I didn't, and then, of course, when Colin done this crime, that was it, they just didn't want to know me. All of them, they just all turned against us. The girls were not really close to their cousins, never seen them very much. It was me mam who kept everyone together and when she died that was it, they just all drifted.

Me dad, I don't know, he does get on with them, but he can be a bit grumpy, you know he's not a grandfather that you would want to be seeing all the time, he's a bit … I don't know … he seems to have a lot of bitterness and I don't know why, but me dad's always been like that. He's not a person you can get really close to, me mam was the one, she kept the family together.

Social services weren't involved until this happened with Colin, that's when it all came out. Oh, they were interested [in what had happened to Louise] after what Colin had done, that's when it all came out, but before that they didn't know, they didn't know none of this. With John, I didn't know who to tell because he was dead; I didn't know what to do. But, after Colin, well, I'll be honest with you, I felt as if they were blaming me for what happened to Louise, I just felt, like, they thought I should have known, I should have seen signs, it was a horrible, a horrible experience. It was just the questions they were asking, trying to get us to explain things and I couldn't do it because I didn't know, I just didn't know what was happening. I was under the doctor, but I seemed to be getting out of that until Colin done this, and then I lost me job, I was on the sick for a lot of months, on the Prozac. They classed it as depression. I can't remember, I honestly can't remember if I did tell him [the GP] what had happened with Louise, I'm not sure. I think I did, I think I would have because me doctor who I went to see, he was very understanding, he would listen to you and I would have told him; I'm sure I would have told him.

The reason I got involved with this [Partners for Protection programme] was after Colin done what he did and it all came out about what had happened with Louise so I had to go and see Stephanie Hill [then consultant psychologist with the Sexual Behaviour Unit] because of the grandson; I had to be capable of looking after the grandson in case Louise didn't get him [if he was removed from her care]. Stephanie Hill said I would benefit. Robert, me new partner, had to go through it as well, but he went through with flying colours. If it hadn't been for Robert, I don't think we would have had Lewis with us, I think he would have been taken away.

I was very, very nervous about coming here; I didn't know what to expect, I didn't want to come and then I thought about it, I thought well, "Is it going to help us? Is it going to benefit us?" So, I did come but they knew how nervous I was because Louise had done it as well before me and she said, "mam, don't worry about it, honestly it's all right, the people are lovely." I did come and I was nervous on the first day but, honestly, it was the best thing I have ever done. It's just opened me eyes to what can happen. It's changed me, it's changed me a lot because I was always very soft with people, I couldn't see no bad in anybody and that's toughened me up, going on this course, I've learnt a lot and that's what I'm saying: I know now what me husband was doing to me, while he was abusing me daughter. It's been really good, it's a really good course to go on. With others like me on the course, it was better for me because I honestly didn't think I would be able to speak out or join in anything because I am very shy and quiet and they couldn't believe it when I said I was quiet, because I wasn't. I shocked meself, but I got on with everybody. All the women were brilliant, really nice, and it was nice for me as well because I lost all me friends and I don't go out anywhere. Me partner does permanent nights and we only get together weekends, so most of the time I've got the grandson, so we don't get any time together, so on that eight-week course it was lovely, really nice, I miss it, I do miss it.

When what happened to Louise, I thought I was the only person who didn't see what was happening in me own family, I couldn't believe that, you know, there was anybody else. I thought I was the only one, but apparently I wasn't – there's a lot of people where things are happening in the family and they don't know. But even then I was still reluctant to talk about the Colin carry-on; I was still scared to disclose anything. I had to do it in a way that they [the course members] wouldn't catch on to who he was [the case had been well publicised]. Before this conviction he had sexually abused a little girl at the swimming bath, that's the bit that I sort of mentioned. I didn't mention the other one because I was scared, I was really scared. I felt like I cheated them, but I had to think of me family now and me grandson because if anyone found out where we were living, Colin has a lot of friends who are eager to get a hold of Louise and they will hurt Lewis, they will hurt the family; they are out to get us because they can't get Colin.

When John was alive, Colin was nowhere near us because his dad wouldn't allow it. His dad kept Colin well away because I think he was scared Colin was going to say things, talk, because Colin was apparently abused by his dad. John just said he was trouble, he would have the police at your door. I'd meet him if he popped round to the house to try and talk to his dad, but his dad would go outside and talk to him and then he would chase him. When he moved in with Louise, that's when I got to know him properly. To be honest with you, I did give him the benefit of the doubt, I thought he had really calmed down, but I didn't know he and Louise were having a relationship, you see, I didn't even know Lewis was Colin's son until Colin had committed the crime. Louise had told us that it was a one night stand and I believed her. Me view of Colin – before it all happened – was that he looked after Louise, but they argued, they did argue a lot and there was a bit of violence which I know about but Louise won't admit to that. She would phone up. "mam, can you come and get Lewis because we have been fighting again," and she didn't want Lewis around when they were fighting. Me partner [Robert] would dash up, get in the car go, pick Lewis up and bring him back, and five minutes later it was as if nothing had happened and this used to go on all the time, me partner used to get really fed up with it and he would say to Louise, "I wish you would just leave him, find somewhere for you and Lewis and just leave him, because it's just not working out." But Louise, no, she didn't see any harm in him. As far as I know, John was really good to him when he was young. He bought him everything he needed, he was good like that.

When Louise got together with him, I thought it has all started again: Louise has gone through a lot and now she has got him she is with an abuser again but the thing was with Colin that there was a lot of allegations about him messing with little boys, different things he had to go to court for but they was "pushed out". I don't know what it's called, it's what they call it when they haven't got enough evidence but there's a lot of them on his record. Social services knew this and they came out to Louise's house because they knew she had a baby in the house and they said everything was fine. There was another man used to go down regular to see Colin – it was something to do with the probation thing but I can't remember his name – and he knew there was a baby in the house and nothing was ever done about that. Yet since all this happened social services said something should have been done, but it wasn't; that Lewis shouldn't have been in the house, he shouldn't have been around Colin. I don't think Colin had ever hurt him, but he shouldn't have been there.

When he committed this other crime [the first allegation against him], I was really annoyed with Louise because she knew he had committed the crime at the swimming baths against this little girl. I says to him, "Colin, what have you done?" he says, "I was in the van, I stopped outside the swimming baths as I wanted the toilet so I dashed out the van, went in, went in the wrong cubicle, there was a girl stood there and I touched her and I ran back out again." And I says, "So why have you had to go to prison and why is the girl saying different?" "I don't know", he says "I don't know. I think she's just trying to cause trouble or something." Anyway that was it, and I finally got the truth that he had done more than that to her. Louise said that that was it, she didn't want nothing more to do with him, but he begged her and begged her and said that he wouldn't do anything ever again, that would be it, that would be the finish, so Louise accepted that.

She said to me that she would give him one chance, and if it ever happened again, that would be it and, of course, he did this other crime [the abduction and abuse] and that was just … well, I just couldn't take no more. At first, to be truthful, I didn't believe that he had done it because I couldn't believe he could have done that, I honestly couldn't believe it, it was such an awful thing to have done. I finally thought about it when the evidence was coming out, and I started to believe it. I thought it must have been him, it had to be him, but I couldn't understand why he went that far, you know, little defenceless girl. I believe it now, one hundred per cent I believe it now.

It took Louise a long time, and eventually she did believe it. It was hard for her, it was really hard. I just kept saying to her, "Louise, you have got to believe it, you have to believe it," and all she would say was, "But mam, it's hard." I says, "I know it's hard," she says "I think a lot of him, I love him." That's what she said, she loved him, he'd done a lot for her, he'd done a lot for Lewis; but I says, "Look, Louise, look what he's done."

Louise's accepted it now. But, of course, she lost her house, all her belongings, they [neighbours] ransacked her house, they broke the doors down and everything, so she had to come out of there, she had to move in with us, which was hard, very hard because she hadn't lived with her parents, she hadn't lived with us, for a long time. She didn't want that but she had no choice, she had no choice. At the time we were living in [name of area] and everything seemed to be all right [after Colin's conviction], apart from cameras, photographers, press constantly on all the time. It was terrible, it was really bad. We got rid of them finally but one day, I think it was one of me daughters went to the shop just at the end of the street, and there's a lamppost with was a poster on it, with all the details about Louise and Colin, where she was living. So we went right round the estate looking for some more posters. They were scattered everywhere, we got them all but we couldn't risk living there any more so we had to phone the police. They came and they had to get us out straight away. We were out the following day I think it was, they had us living in Amble, they had us living in a hotel in the town, they had us living in Gateshead, and, finally, where we are now, so there's been a lot of upheaval. I'm very annoyed with Colin, I blame him for all this, I really do. I don't want to see him, I don't even want to speak to him. He thinks Louise wants nothing to do with him because of the social services, he thinks they're stopping her but little does he know Louise wants nothing more to do with him full stop. She is going to get an order out stopping him from even trying to contact Lewis. I don't even know where he is now because he was moved from his first prison.

It was Christmas Eve 2006 and Colin went out, Louise was bathing Lewis and she didn't know where he had gone because he was always popping in and out. He said he came back in because he had forgotten something but at that time he was meant to have come back in, this was when it was meant to have happened. He came back that night without his coat, so where was his coat, where did he leave his coat? He must have used that – that's all I keep thinking – he has used that to wrap the girl up.

The problem was the court case was in Newcastle Crown Court and we could see it from where we were living, but we couldn't go out because there was cameras around. We were convinced that somebody knew where we were living, because there was always somebody down at the bottom, near where the Millennium Bridge starts, with this massive big camera, like a TV thing. We were scared to go out on them days because we couldn't go past the court or nothing, because all his mates were there making sure that he was going to get locked up, or trying to get to him but we were petrified.

Yes, it could very well have been, it could very well have been [that Louise didn't want to think this could happen twice over to her]. It was hard for Louise to talk about her abuse because she hadn't had any counselling and it was still inside her and it was so hard for her to talk about it. We are quite close, but she does tend to hold a lot of things back, she's very deep. She came here [to Partners for Protection] because of what happened, because she was living with Colin, an abuser, and they thought she shouldn't have been because she was putting Lewis at risk. She was but she couldn't see that, she couldn't see Colin touching Lewis – do you know what I mean? – because he had never done nothing to Lewis: she used to bathe him, she changed his nappy and everything. Colin was never, like, connected to Lewis that way because he was hardly ever in; he was in and out all the time. She done everything for Lewis, but they kept saying to her, "What would happen if he was in and Lewis was downstairs and you had to go the toilet?" I never thought about that you know, how quick it could happen.

Do you know, that's a sore point about when Lewis gets older? We just don't know how we're going to do it [to tell him]. It's going to be really hard. What our worry is – well my worry – is if anybody finds out Lewis's connection, who his dad is. For a little while he would ask where his dad was and Louise would just say, "Daddy's working away, son, he's working on the cars," and he would accept that but for a while he hasn't really asked, so we are just hoping it's going to stay like that. But he's a very, very clever, very bright little boy for his age, but, in the future, I don't know how we are going to explain to him because he's going to ask, and it's going to be very hard, very hard.

With Louise having to move into the family home again, it's been quite difficult, we've had our ups and downs, we seem to be clashing ... more so because of Lewis, like who is in charge of him and he has got three adults telling him all different messages. He knows who to go to to be petted up and get what he wants – that's me. His mam's very strict, he knows he can't get away with nothing with his mam. His granda's a bit soft with him and he's not used to being told off by his granda and when he does get told off by his granda, he cries because he thinks, "Well, Granda you don't usually tell me off," but if he does something really bad he does get told off. It has been difficult because with three adults (and I've got the other daughter, Marie, she's 20, she's living at home) and it is hard, it is hard and they haven't got no privacy really, with Louise's used to being in her own house.

Me other daughter, Dawn, didn't want nothing to do with Colin, nothing at all, but she's very soft, she takes after me there and he was phoning her from the prison because he got her phone number. He was phoning Louise but Louise got told by social services she had got to have no contact with him but it was hard to get him to stop phoning. He kept on phoning Dawn and Dawn was too soft to say, "Colin, I don't want you ringing us," so I got on to social services and told them that he was ringing Dawn and they told me to tell her to get on to the prison to get her number taken off and that's the way we had to do it. It was also causing problems with Dawn and her partner because he hated Colin for what he'd done, and it was upsetting Dawn because she didn't want to speak to Colin.

Marie and Louise are very, very close. They work together. Dawn, she's got her own place with her boyfriend, they've got a little girl. She's pregnant again. She keeps herself to herself, and her and Louise don't really get on at the minute but they'll speak. I think it could be because of what Louise was told – to get away from Colin – and I think Dawn blames Louise for the break-up of the family, having to move away. I think Dawn blames her because Louise shouldn't have been with him.

How do I look at life? Well, I'll be honest with you – I just want to have a happy life now and in the future, I just don't want anything to go wrong ever again, because this has destroyed the whole family, it has, it's broke the whole family up. I've lost me sister, I've lost me brothers, me dad (I hardly speak to him), I've got no friends now, I've only got me partner, who's brought Lewis up from the beginning, who has been there for us, through all this from when me husband died, he was there right the way through. I've felt guilty for him, because he's had to go through all this and he shouldn't have, you know, he shouldn't have been involved in it, and we lost the house.

I think Dawn was upset because we've had to move away and we'd lived next to Dawn. She still lives down there [where they lived as a family] and she doesn't get no problems now; she did in the beginning but she is all right now. I think she was more upset because it took me away from near her, you know, which is understandable; it broke the whole family. I'm still angry now with Colin, really am angry – why he done it and what trouble he's caused this family. It's unbelievable.

It would probably have been better if I'd been able to talk about Colin in the [Partners for Protection] group, probably, but I couldn't, it was too dangerous. Don't get us wrong: they probably wouldn't have, but you see, they could have gone out, talked to their friends, and that would get back to somebody else and you know, I just couldn't do it, I would have loved to talk about it, I really would. No one's really said anything about seeing a counsellor but I feel like this course has helped me an awful lot, it really has: I am a changed person – I'm not as scared to do anything any more. I came here today to see you, bright as a button, I wasn't nervous or nothing and I would have been before all this. I was never a one to mingle in, like, group discussions; very shy, I couldn't speak out. I have always been the same, I feel like everybody's … if you're going to say something, everybody's going to look at you and I felt, I don't know, I just feel, it's a funny feeling but I feel fine now.

I can speak out now, I've got a lot more confidence, I can look after me grandson and me other grandchildren. I'll be there to look after them and if I see any sign at all, that'll be it. I don't want them to go through what Louise's gone through, especially Lewis. It's going to be hard enough for him when he gets older, knowing what his dad's done and that his dad could be potentially his uncle. It's, you know, not nice, not nice at all, so how's he going to react towards me and his mam?

Karen Williams

"You need to do something with your life – change it"

Karen Williams is 23 and comes from a family where there is a long history of sexual abuse. What she learned about her partner, Ross Browning, may have awakened in her much of her past. Her grandfather abused her. He had also abused one of her aunts, who then abused Karen's father, who, in turn, abused one of his sisters. Emotionally abused by both her mother, who is 42, and father, who is 50, Karen was also sexually abused by two cousins on different sides of her family from the age of 4 until she was taken into care at 12. She was also abused by other men in whose care she was left by her parents while they went drinking. She received counselling at Mosaic when in care and she retains a strong and supportive relationship with her former foster carer, Mary. She has little, if anything, to do with her family.

She is a lively member of the Partners for Protection group, always ready to speak up, and occasionally she adopts the language of therapy. When members of her group are asked if they would volunteer to be interviewed for this book, she agrees immediately, even very enthusiastically. The others decline. When she is interviewed, she is forthcoming but more measured in her behaviour. While all the interviewees say how much they learned from their work on the Parents for Protection course, Karen makes a point of being specific about how this applies also to other matters – for example, her worry as to why Gavin, her 9-year-old brother, displays sexualised behaviour. The course appears, too, to have allowed her to make some sense of her life.

Karen lived with Ross Browning, whom she met when she was nearly 16. He was 17, a man with dyslexia, a mild learning disability, and other disabilities. He, too, had been in care and his mother had drug and alcohol problems. She was pregnant with their first child, Zoë, 1, when she found out that her partner had previously sexually abused his cousin and they ceased to live together. However, despite that, she became pregnant by him again with Ashley, who is 7 months old. Karen has no idea where Ross is now. Zoë went into care in January 2007 and Ashley went into care when she was two days old. Karen lives on benefits but has worked for GNER, the former rail company, and on the shop-floor of a supermarket. She now says that she wants to work where she can help people. One day, too, she says, she hopes to write a book about her life.

I was brought in a pretty much violent household with me mam and dad. There was a lot of alcohol, a lot of aggression, and a lot of me parents leaving me unsupervised with adults that they didn't really know too well. On both me dad's side and me mam's side of the family I was abused by family members. It was both me cousins and a baby-sitter from a pub next to where me dad used to go drinking on a regular basis, and it continued again another three or four times by different people due to again me dad ... well, both parents leaving me unsupervised while they were out socialising and concentrating on alcohol. It began when I was 4 and went on right through until I was placed in care when I was 12.

It wasn't just that reason I was taken into care: me dad used to emotionally abuse me and when he had given up on that, then me mam used to then take over his role of emotionally abusing me as well. At the time, I suppose I would have been very confused, not knowing why it was happening; I think I've pretty much spent me life very confused.

I didn't realise how common [child sexual abuse] was: I realised it happened, but obviously I didn't like know the percentage of how many men abuse children, I wasn't, like, one hundred per cent on that.

I left care when I was 18 and when I was, I think, 16, I went into full-time education because I was brought out of school when I was 14, so I didn't like get any of me GCSEs or nothing that I needed so I then went on to education to gain the GCSEs that I needed. Then I moved into me own flat and then I worked for GNER until I was 19 and then I fell pregnant with me daughter, and well, I've been with me partner, well, me ex-partner, since I was 15 so I would have just been turning on 16 when I met him. Me relationship with him broke up when I was pregnant with Ashley. It would have been January last year [2007]. I met him in college.

It was a normal relationship, yes. At the very beginning when I had first met him, he was very bubbly, very happy, but he was also a very quiet person as well. I think in them days when you are like ... well even still now ... when you meet young people of that age, you know, you find men are very immature and get themselves into trouble, whereas he was the opposite and he didn't get involved in any trouble, he stayed away from it and I suppose that's what I liked about him. He didn't come across like other men and I saw that as a decent person. I thought that we would get married and have children.

His mam was or still is, even to this day, very much into drug substances, and she abuses alcohol and she can be quite violent in her tone when she has had a lot to drink and uses drugs. His mam was, like, a lesbian. She had that partner there, Joanie; she was also the same or still is very much an alcoholic. I don't think Joanie associates with drugs as much as his mam does, but they're pretty much the same. I didn't have a lot of access to his family really because he was very isolated from his family and he didn't tend to associate too much with his mam or if and when he did, it was a very negative attitude what he would get off his family.

It was pretty exciting when I fell pregnant [with Zoë]. I was looking forward to having a daughter of me own, and I think as far as me ex-partner was concerned he had pretty much had mixed feelings about the fact that I was pregnant and I kind of understand why now because of his own past. Obviously, at the time I didn't know anything about his past, nothing was disclosed. I think the only time at that point what I did know was that he had a lot of disabilities. He was dyslexic, you pretty much had to motivate him to do things, like housework or maybe just go out and pay a bill, go shopping. You had to give him that push. Well, I didn't judge him, I wasn't judgemental because of his disabilities and I didn't see that as a sign of him abusing the child. I did, however, see it as he had a lot of problems in the past because he was also in care himself. I thought it was pretty much down to the fact that his mam was on drugs and I didn't realise it was because he had abused his own family member.

I found out about that when I fell pregnant with Zoe. When you've got to go for check-ups at the doctors and while you're pregnant, the midwife obviously got this information of who I was with and she then obviously had to pass it on to social services. Then there was social workers involved, plus I had me leaving care worker as well (she was another person who found out about his past).

I'm pretty much assuming that they found out by checking records. We were all sat down in, like, a conference room and at this time I didn't have an understanding as to what was going on and then the social worker and the manager of social services sat me down and said for Ross to tell me that he would have to explain to me why social services became involved.

Then I was told the information that when he was 14 he had abused his cousin, and I think at that time I didn't really know how to think or how to take it because I had been with him for such a long time and then to find out years later down the line that's what he had done as a teenager was a big shock, plus knowing that I'd been there and been through that.

He was saying that he was sorry, and he didn't mean for this all to come out and he didn't want it to come out. He didn't want to tell us because he knew about me past because I had told him and he was scared how I would react when I found out about his past. He said that he was very naive as a child, he didn't understand, he thought that he was doing … he wasn't doing anything wrong, and he hated himself for what he had done and it was the worst mistake he could ever have made and that he would never harm another child again. He believes that people that harm children are sick – that was the terms and words he used, that the adults are sick for doing that to children.

It brought a lot of … it surfaced a lot of me past, and it made me sort of sit in her [Ross's cousin's] shoes, remembering what I felt like, what she must have felt like. I was thinking about things like that and the confusion that that little girl must have went through at the time. I felt uncomfortable, very uncomfortable. I felt out of place and it, like, brought a lot of my past back when I was told about this and I automatically felt very mixed up, confused straight away. I just didn't … I was stuck, I didn't know what to do.

Then Ross had to go for an SBU [Sexual Behaviour Unit] assessment [in Newcastle] to see at that stage what risk he was. I don't know if it came back that he was a medium risk or a low one, but they then had more meetings with me on a regular basis, without Ross's presence, to basically find out if I was able to protect me child and then we had a final conference when Zoë was born. The social services then were happy that Ross could gradually have unsupervised contact with me daughter and they also believed that I was capable enough of protecting my child from me ex-partner.

I was pregnant with Ashley, but I also realised that I was taking on a lot of work with Ross and a lot of depression overtook me and I sort of forgot the outside of me sort of thing, I forgot everybody around us, and started to forget who I was at that time, even though social services said that they were fine that Ross had unsupervised contact. I then became quite aggressive towards Ross afterwards, not physically, just very verbal and I became very paranoid and, like, it got to the point where I had to take Zoë to the bathroom with us because I wouldn't leave her. I'd put something under me bedroom door because I didn't want him sleeping in the same bedroom while Zoë was in the cot because I was frightened in case he came in and done something to her. When I was cooking she had to come into the kitchen with us and it became that all the time and it became so straining because I had no help and I had nobody around to help me to like ... while I had to take care of Ross's disabilities and his needs and then also Zoë, then keeping on top of the housework and things that needed doing, but then once me depression got worse me home conditions started to slip.

I decided enough was enough. I needed to change me life, but also then social services realised the condition of me ill-health and asked Ross to move out of the house. They were pretty shocked to see the state I was in, but I didn't see it at the time, I was poorly; everybody around us did but me, so I was kind of in denial of being poorly at the time.

The depression was about having me past, but also carrying the burden of Ross, knowing what he had done, carrying the burden of having to protect me daughter, having to look after Ross and his disabilities all the time, having to make sure he's never alone. I think then I became a loner and isolated. I had nobody that I could turn to for support at the time or I didn't want to turn to anybody for support.

I've got two brothers but I don't have contact with them. Me younger brother, Gavin, who is 9, I see him from time to time but he also displays a lot of sexualised behaviour, so I tend to distance meself from that because it's a concern to me where and how he's got this sexualised behaviour, where it's coming from. It's making me think that something's happened to him, or he's watched something on TV because he's got a TV in his bedroom and me mam let's him watch TV out of hours and I believe that he could be noticing or witnessing things on there also. But there is no way of knowing and I just kind of keep out of it and leave that job to social services, because I know it's their job and it is up to them to do that. They did have involvement but the supervision is now over but they haven't really gone anywhere with finding out why Gavin is doing what he's doing.

Me other brother, he'll be 22 coming up. He's a drug user, he's very violent. He's been arrested on numerous occasions, he's spent a short while on remand in custody, so that's another reason I tend not to have too much to do with any of the family because the history.

I came back [to Mosaic] because I had to go for an SBU assessment. They were happy at the beginning with me as a parent. I spent a short time in a women's refuge and at the time I was suffering still from a lot of depression and I was pregnant. I was at the refuge because me ex-partner kept coming back to me home, he kept like turning up, saying he had nowhere to go and he had no one to stay with. Then that pretty much got on top of me, because I knew what was at risk by him keep coming back so then I got social services to help us move from where I was living into the women's refuge and that was one of the worst mistakes I could ever have made. It was horrible in there. They were bullies. I know the women in there have also come from bad backgrounds but I kind of believed at the time when you come from a bad background and you've been abused or hurt in any way shape of form, you wouldn't, therefore, do it to anybody else. When I was there I chose to wash the floor, and they would purposely spill coffee all over so I would have to clean it up again and then you had your own fridge and they would go in there while I wasn't there and take all me food, so I was pretty much bullied in there. I was kept pretty much meself and I didn't really associate with the group. I kind of stayed away from it after a while.

Me younger brother came and stayed at the refuge for a night's stay and there was an incident where all the young children were left in the playroom in there. They had all taken part on this little girl of, like, touching her and touching her privates, they all took part in it. Then after that, that's why the SBU then became back involved again because the social services said I would then need to be re-assessed for that same thing and then they decided I needed to be sent on to this [Partners for Protection] course.

The doctor [who did the second assessment] recommended that me children were returned home to me, and even though this was suggested, it didn't happen. I don't think it was all or so much to do with me problems; it was everybody else around me, it's like I was stuck in the middle of everybody else's past and everybody else's problems and it got too much.

I think, if I remember, even at the beginning of this, I was kind of thinking, "Well do I attract child abusers? Do I seem vulnerable because of me own past?" That's what I did think because of me past. And then I was thinking, "Why have you got to meet somebody else the same, that's done the same to what happened to me as a child, another child abuser?" And it's like, then I started to think, "How do you know like who's a child abuser?" How can you work this out in your own head because you can meet the nicest person in the world and then they turn out that that's what happens. But looking back over the last eight weeks of this course [the day of the interview was Karen's last day on the course], it's made me realise and sort of helped me to understand that child abuse is very planned and in a child abuser's eyes it takes a lot of work for how he can get from one place to abusing a child.

Men can be very, very manipulating and very convincing and it's just ... it's crazy, but looking at somebody else's life like a map sort of thing, of how many children has been abused and where it all fits in, you can see the wider picture. But it gets quite frustrating when the other person can't see that. Like, it's the same with me ex-partner. I did say to the girls in the group, "Is it really worth sticking with your ex-partner or partner to wait around if he is a child abuser? Is it really worth the risk that your children could then be abused? Is it worth taking that risk? Because I don't believe it is."

It makes me very wary about meeting people again in the future. I know that if I do ever meet men in the future I'm going to be more aware of it, but I'm going to be looking out more, even more for the signs that are there, of how they can get from motivation to looking at their past. It's pretty much going to be doing a lot of questioning, if I do step into another relationship again. It will be a very long time before I ever have another relationship and do allow another person next to me children but obviously I know that not everybody's like that and there is some genuine people out there.

You do sometimes think [of a friendly stranger], "Why is he smiling at me for? Why is he looking at me like that?" or "What way is he looking at us? Is he looking at us in just a normal genuine way? Is he looking at me in a way, like a provocative sexual way or is he attracted to me?"

I would hope that I will have brought me daughters up enough to understand that you don't talk to strangers and you don't go anywhere near strangers, you stay next to me all the time. I do want to make them aware of strangers. Zoë was very attached to me, and she had good attachment because she was very shy where other people were concerned, she would stay right next to the adult that she was with and she wouldn't go anywhere near the person, or the strange person. I sort of pretty much put that down to the fact that was how I had brought me daughter up, even though she is so young at the moment. Me and her had such a strong bond. She knows that strange people are strange people basically, but as far as men, like, smiling at me daughter, I don't want her to like feel that a person's bad for smiling at you. I would be more concerned as to what kind of look or what way he was looking at me daughter; that's when I would think about it more.

I have never ever hated social services because I've been there throughout me life with social services, so I'm always getting on with them, but I did feel at one point I was treated very unfairly. I didn't get on with me social worker because she was never there when I needed to speak to her, or she was always on the sick. She spent half her life on the sick so I couldn't never get in touch with her if I needed her help, she would never come out and see me or let me know the progress. I know she's me children's social worker but also she has to communicate with me in order for me to put things right if she believes I'm doing something wrong. I think everybody, as far as the court, was getting pretty hacked off with me social worker because me children were supposed to be back three or four weeks ago, but because she's spent so much time on the sick it slowed things down.

The police didn't become involved at all. I think the only time they were ever about was at [case] conferences. There was a police officer to make sure that there was no reports that anything had happened, no violent attacks or anything like that, or anything had gone on in me home.

I really believe that both me mam and dad are very naive, I think they're very … they haven't got any understanding of child abuse and feel that it's normal. I had a lot of emotional abuse from me dad when I was abused. He spent a lot of years saying it was my fault, like from me past and that I was a slag, that I caused it. I was the one that made them go out on the drink. Then they put me with baby-sitters, me cousins, and I think I was abused a lot of times by a lot of different men because of the result of me mam and dad not protecting me properly. When me dad said it was me fault, he then would start to feel guilty and say it wasn't me fault. Then me mam would take over that role of me dad and say it was me fault, and so they sort of both played mind games.

I had no respect for either of them once I did mature because when I went into care, it was the best thing because that abuse just stopped, it wasn't happening any more, it was like something had just disappeared from me life and it was all the hurt and the pain and … I did go from placement to placement for a while. I went into a few different places until they then found me a full-time carer which is who I still see now. I first went into care when I was 12 and I think it must have been about – if I can remember that far back – it must have been about 12 months after that when I eventually went into that placement.

I can't remember how I came about disclosing [to my parents] the abuse that had happened to me, but I know what did happen is that once they did find out it took two years before they said anything about the first abuse, two years to get the police involved. I think it was a nurse who I told at the school and I think the head teacher became involved and then the police became involved. I think me parents were both in denial that anything had ever happened to me. Then it was too late for anything to happen to one of me cousins and there was only ever three men that were sentenced.

I was abused by me granddad and that was the one abuse I didn't disclose – me granddad had passed away – because I thought I had been through so much, like the amount of abuse I suffered, and none of the family ever believed anything had happened to us, none of me aunties, or anything. So much of me family was saying it was my fault, that none of these abusers have done anything wrong. It was all down to me, I was telling lies. I kind of got to the point where I was just sick, because I had been abused that many times and it felt like I was just in no end of abuse and I didn't want to go through all the video links [for court appearances] again and all the medical examinations. I just had enough.

None of me family know that me granddad had abused us apart from Mary, me ex-foster carer, but she knows herself there wouldn't have been anything they could have done now because me granda's dead. It was only about a month ago I went and walked all over his grave. I got the bus to Lemington, where they're from, and I went to the graveyard and stamped all over it. I was going through a lot of hurt because of me children and then I had memories of my past and had hatred for me ex-partner because of what he had put us through. For some reason I kept seeing me granddad's face. It was like, when I was walking in the passageway, the hallway of me home, I would turn and I would see me granddad out of the blue for no reason and I just thought the only way to go and get rid of him was to go and walk all over his grave and just hope that he would never enter me head again which I knew he probably would. When I did it I felt a lot better. I mean, I swore at the grave. I was there for about half an hour standing on the grave. I must have looked like a nutter to whoever walked past but it made me feel better. I just wanted to leave me past in his grave, I wanted to leave it with him.

I know this won't happen to me children, I won't ever let it happen to me children because when I look back at how horrible me life was and the torture I suffered through me family and the memories I still hold now, it just makes me protect me children even more from me family and any other person for that matter. I suppose that's why I was the way I was when I heard like Ross's past. I just thought, "You're not going to get that chance to do anything to me children." I won't leave me children unsupervised with anybody. I think there is only one stable person I will ever trust with me children and that's me ex-foster carer; other than that I don't trust anybody with me children. Even now, at the minute, with them being in care, it worries us every day because I still think I don't know these foster carers. Yes, they can be professionals but you still hear of people like that abusing children and it runs through my head every day. I have got social services reassuring me, saying that this won't happen and I'm always saying, "Well, how do you know?" and they say they have been police checked and I say, "Well, people that have abused can be police checked and it won't ever come out."

Ross never attended any of his court cases that he's supposed to attend for contact with Zoë and Ashley, which is a good thing really. Well, I'm pretty much pleased about it because I don't believe he's got any parenting skills, plus his past and plus I've told social services that there's no way on this earth that I would be taking part in supervising contacts. I didn't want any part of that because I didn't want him to believe that he could have a chance of getting back as a family. I wanted him to believe it was over and I didn't want that stress of having to supervise contact. I believed that if [social services] thought I said that I would prefer he didn't see the children but if they believe that that's what he needs to do, it's up to them to take over the supervision, not me.

I do have a lot better understanding of Ross [having been on the Partners for Protection course], looking at the motivation side of things like his background, where he's come from, the things that happened to him. I do have an understanding, but also looking back at me, I've suffered more abuse and I haven't turned out to be like that, 'cos I had a lot of help. He's not received any help at all, all's I know is he did have treatment, like prevention, but as far as counselling to talk about it, I don't think he's ever had that.

I did hate him because he'd deceived me and of what he'd done and knowing what I had been through, the fact that he could do that to a child. Looking back, once I've done this course and it's over, I don't hate him, but I kind of, like, pity him in a way because he's got the rest of his life to go with the way he is now with his disabilities. He's got no help because MENCAP [the charity for people with a learning disability] haven't become involved, so he's got nobody to help him. But I kind of believe that he's at the stage of his life where he is now for a reason. His life now – what would it be? What I can imagine it to be is lonely, without anybody in his life. It happens for a reason. I believe because of what he's done, he's being punished for it.

Me? I want more out of me life; I don't want to be just behind the till for the rest of me life, working in a shop. I want to do something where I can afford to take care of me children and they can have good futures, go to university, do things that they want to do. I want to encourage them to become somebody themselves; that's what I want to do. There's a lot of things I want to do out me life now and I know I can do it. If I stick me mind to something I can do it and I know I have got the brains to do that. I'm kind of into forensic science – the criminal side of forensic science – also death, murders and stuff like that, and I like history but I also want to write a book.

I don't so much say it's the professionals that have helped me to decide what I want to do. I think it's looking at other people's lives, backgrounds and how difficult it is for other people; I would also like to go into helping other people. It's life's experiences that has made us want to really do something like this with me future. Yeah, to go for that because me ex-foster carer, she said she could really see me doing something where I'm helping other people, but she did say, "I think at the minute you have had so much going on in your life you haven't had a chance to live your own life, i.e., like your childhood was lost, and it was taken from you, so people just want to see you happy and living what you missed out on them years ago." But I still would like to help other people, and I would also like to help other people with abuse because I know I've suffered it and I have come through it. I would like to be able to have that impact on somebody else. I was pleased at the end of the group 'cos I had a card written to us by all the group saying that I've helped them learn a lot from this course from the things that I've said to them.

Both Shelagh [Scott, senior practitioner, Mosaic] and Richard [Jackson, senior practitioner, Mosaic] have said that I've done extremely well on the course and I've worked hard. I know I've worked hard at what I've done and I'm glad that I've been able to be an inspiration to other people.

I think there was only one person I wasn't an inspiration to [in the group] because I think she was in a frame [of mind] and still is now. I don't believe this course has helped her as she is still stuck in denial and doesn't believe that her partner has done anything. Last Monday I got very upset. I had mixed feelings and was very angry but I got up and walked out of the room rather than blow me top because I would never do that, I would never make anybody feel uncomfortable because I believe that that's their past. It was when they read the story to us about one of the women's pasts. It was very graphical but she [the other group member] still didn't believe it, that this 3-year-old had been abused by her partner and it made me pretty angry because what was described was what happened to me.

Me own life experience sort of brought me to realise where I am with me life, where I want to be with me future and me children and I sort of gained a lot of experience from me ex-foster carer because I see her a lot; she's very much a support to me and she's even asked herself if she could have adopted me. She would have and she's been there pretty much all my support and I think I really came sane through just a lot of life experience.

Looking back on me own life over the last 23 years I have been through a lot to get where I am today. I'm proud that I have been able to get this far because, I guess, at the beginning I kind of believed, or sort of put it into me own head, that I wasn't going to get anywhere in me life, it was just going to get worse, and I got to the situation where it was, "Why is it keep happening to me for? What am I doing so wrong to make me life so bad?" and I think all that just fitted into, "You need to do something with your life – change it."

Rachel Bond

"Tom is a good person who's done a very bad thing"

Rachel Bond is 41 and, with her husband, Tom, she has two children, Mark, aged 7, and Sarah, aged 5. She works for a charity. At the time of being interviewed (November 2007), Rachel was looking forward to Tom returning to live with them as a family in their home in a small town in Lancashire, after serving 16 months of his 32-month sentence for downloading child pornography from the internet. He had been released in September 2007. She tells her story articulately and calmly until she comes to describe how she learned of her husband's crime. At one point, she is very obviously distressed and tearful. Tom has two adult children, Matthew, 27, and Beth, 23, by his previous marriage, who, while they have contact with their mother, have also shared a home, as children, with their father and Rachel.

I would say my childhood was very happy and very stable. My parents divorced when I was 7 or 8. My mother was fantastic. She remarried when I was 8, so there was a period of time when she was going out with my stepfather, but really we were on our own. I have a brother who is a year younger than me. My gran lived nearby and that was our family. My mother worked very, very hard to have a job which perhaps didn't challenge her as much as she would have liked, to keep things together. She was a very good parent. My dad kept in touch but he moved down to Norfolk initially and then to New Zealand, so we kept in touch but obviously it's a fair old distance so the contact there wasn't as much as I would have liked, but I don't have any doubt that he loved us. Keeping in touch with us was not as he would have wished it to have been but probably he made the best of bad circumstances. Neither of them is alive.

There's another crisis in all of this, just how events have a tendency to sort of come together. Tom was assaulted when he was out one evening, and ended up with this head injury and we didn't know what the outcome was going to be, but my mother was in the hospital having a tumour removed from the area round her heart, so it was incredibly stressful. Really, that was when we saw her health decline. From that point she had to go through this huge operation and then obviously had to have chemotherapy and radiotherapy and the site of the tumour was associated with this neurological condition called myokymia. Although she recovered in steps from the various things, her health generally declined and Tom and I moved from where we had been living to our present house, five years ago so. That would have been in the summer of 2002. My dad had died the year before my mum, very unexpectedly. She died in December 2002 and Sarah was born in September 2002. The knock on the door was in May 2004.

Mark was born in June 2000 and I was taking him across to New Zealand to visit Dad in the September. He came across to visit us because he'd turned 65 in the January 2001 and I helped him sort out his UK pension. Then he came across again in Easter that year and he had only been home a matter of weeks and he dropped dead.

Tom and I met in 1990 on a course and we sort of kept in touch and commuted for probably about a year after that. Then we had to think about who would be best off moving if we were to be together and he ended up moving up to this area. I had a flat at the time so Tom moved in with me – we got married in 1998 – and then we sold his house and the flat and bought a house together. Very quickly after that he was quite seriously assaulted and pensioned out the fire service. He sustained a really severe head injury and so all the plans you have for how things are going to be rapidly disintegrated. The first year after the assault was a bit of a write-off really because he was very poorly. His skull fracture wasn't initially diagnosed, but as a result of that he was diagnosed as having epilepsy, which obviously had an effect on driving and all sorts of things so it was really quite isolating. He had moved up and was away from family, friends and work contacts and although everybody around him at work were very, very good it was very, very difficult.

After about a year his condition had settled down enough and really out of a desire to do something and not vegetate, he did an access course and really found an interest in law, decided he'd like to be a solicitor (taking on criminal and other cases rather than conveyancing) and saw that as a way for him to progress a career path, and he worked very, very hard. When we'd met he had a fantastic memory – I'd never really met anybody with a near-photographic memory before – and then the assault had the effect of ... you know, he would walk from one room to another and not be able to remember what he had gone for, and he lost the ability to count numbers. He has had to work really, really hard to keep things in, so he worked very hard in his access course and he was really well supported by the staff. One particular person acted as a mentor and pushed him, encouraged him to think about a degree course, so he applied for that and did a three-year degree in law. We had a really, really good relationship. He's a bright articulate, funny, hard-working, vulnerable bloke, and I think that incident at that time put a massive strain on things and it's continued in different ways.

The difficulties which affected him have affected us in very practical terms, like him not being able to drive when the kids were young. His head injury was very demoralising. Tom had moved up here with lots and lots of very specialist skills in the fire service and had undertaken a bit of a sacrifice in that he was now going back to working on the front-line – he had had a senior management job – and would do a year kind of to prove himself up here. None of that got to materialise and then your much-loved career is just taken away from you because of somebody's cruelty and stupidity … well, it affected him. He's a big, strapping bloke, a very able bloke and he had basically been pounded and had his head stood on.

It was very demoralising and affected our relationship. Everything took time to overcome, he sort of picked up and as his confidence grew, I think, as he was able to progress and demonstrate his abilities through his very, very hard work on his degree course and that was some compensation. But the outcome was all very uncertain, obviously he didn't know what kind of calibre he was going to be able to achieve and, given the level of competition, what he was going to be able to do at the end of things. I think, as well, that the fact that I was still doing my job, which was pretty responsible, didn't help. Neither of us could do much about it, probably. I suppose he was envious, in some respects, because I did exactly the same sort of things that he had been very capable of doing and the opportunity to do that was no longer there for him. But after the access course and the degree, he took a vocational course which had been put out to the provinces and so he was able to do that up here, so that was a further year. He kind of joined the treadmill of so many people applying for a limited number of places and fortunately he got one.

That somewhat balanced the relationship. I don't want to make it sound as if this was the case all the time but, you know, I was envious of him. Very drastic circumstances enable you to think perhaps of doing something like going to university as an adult and it was a fantastic opportunity so I think that I definitely did feel envious of some of that and I think it was a change from us having a fair idea of our lives and careers progressing in tandem to, you know, taking, not completely different courses but certainly not the life we had seen, the one you maybe map out. He worked just so hard and was consumed by this new career.

I was very, very happy in my career and have had fantastic opportunities to do various things, often working in specialised areas. I had been in the job for 17 years before I left and had Mark. Tom had been in the fire service for 12 years before he had to be medically retired (it might be a little longer than that).

I always wanted children and the children were planned. I was 33 when I had Mark and had seen lots of my girlfriends struggle to work shifts and try to be all things to all people and I don't honestly think that you can do that. You are very lucky if you get things over the course of a lifetime, you can't have it all at once, so it was deliberate. I had the choice: I could have taken a career break but I think I knew I wouldn't want to go back. My mother was very ill, so having family around to help with childcare wasn't really an option and that was always very clear. So it was a deliberate decision not to work after Mark arrived.

When I learned about what Tom had done, I think surprise has to be the gravest understatement. It was a complete, a complete shock. It was May, a beautiful, sunny May morning. Mark had gone off to nursery, Sarah was a baby in arms and I can remember I had got her dressed to play outside in the garden and bimbo around with her on a mat. I was dressed in the tattiest pair of shorts and a T-shirt and just was idyllically happy and then there were two officers from the child protection unit knocking on the door and asking to come in. They then started to explain the circumstances of their concern about the computer. It wasn't to do with the operation [Operation Ore, a high-profile police operation to crack down on users of internet child pornography], but it was obviously a contact from another computer elsewhere in the country to Tom's web address and I was just absolutely stunned, you know. I don't think I have ever experienced shock like it, I couldn't ... I found it difficult to breathe, it was as if he'd been kind of turned to stone, it was ... and the only ... It might make more sense if I asked them to repeat it again. "Can you just say that again?" and again and again and it was just ... it couldn't possibly be, it couldn't possibly be, Tom had ... I can remember thinking just things like ... Well, he had literally just got his first trial [as a solicitor] and there was stuff on the computer about that. I asked them things about security and the documentation and it made absolutely no sense whatsoever, the words made sense but it was just ... I was stunned beyond belief. The computer was seized.

I remember ringing him while they were there and he was absolutely stunned, but was tied up with court. The conversation didn't really go round to ... It wasn't, "Is there any truth in this?" I didn't ask him those questions then, it's just that he was absolutely shocked and I was asking when was he going to be able to get home. Obviously, the computer was going to be looked at and that was when they asked me, "Can we get anybody to come and sit with you?" and I thought, "Who on earth are you going ask? How can you explain this?" and I was just in absolute ... and I didn't want to because I didn't know what to say. Who can you ask? I had to go and collect Mark from nursery quite quickly afterwards. I remember walking down the street on automatic pilot because you have got things to do as a mum and just being absolutely numb. The whole time in the street I was just feeling like an alien really, but on automatic pilot to collect the child, take the child home and Beth, my step-daughter, was living with us at the time. She was at 6th-form college, she had the A-levels coming up within weeks and she had a driving test within days.

I can't remember the dates, I don't know what day of the week, but this was not too far away from Bank Holiday weekend at the end of May, so I think somehow we managed to scrape through the remainder of the week. I had various conversations with Tom about what on earth could all this be about and he made various sorts of admissions to pornography websites and chat-rooms – I don't think I understand yet what a chatroom is – and just being absolutely furious with him about what all this could possibly be about and he didn't ... he wasn't ... Although he had kind of moved towards admitting some involvement in pornography and websites, chatrooms, he hadn't been ... I knew he hadn't been completely honest with me. I just asked him, "How do we sort this out?" How can we sort this out if he can't talk to me? Who can he talk to, because we can't just stay like this? So, over the course of that Bank Holiday weekend we arranged for him to go and see somebody who he thought very highly of, the senior partner in the [law] firm, who had acted as a kind of mentor to him.

He went off to talk to this friend of ours and I think that he probably was more open and honest with him. I think it was after that that he took himself off and didn't come back one day after work. He had a mobile phone and I had been used to being able ring him at lunchtimes and whenever, but there was no contact, I couldn't get through. He'd said he was at a particular court and when I became concerned later in the day, I rang his office and he hadn't been in court, which was even more alarming. Then it got to teatime and he just kind of disappeared. I ended up having to ring somebody else who he had mentioned seeing in the day and I don't know what he thought; I think he thought he had to reassure me that Tom really did love us. Maybe he thought that perhaps Tom was having an affair or something like that, but Tom had disappeared. He had last been seen in Manchester. I had told a couple of my girlfriends about it, and one of them was good enough to go and trawl the car parks in the canal area in Manchester.

It got to between ten and eleven at night and I thought, "Well, what do I do now? Do I report him missing from home and that kind of has the effect of you have to admit the reality of it: 'Why has he?'" But what are the consequences going to be if you don't? But, then you think, "Right, if this has happened because there is an element of truth about it and the bottom line is: do I want him sitting with a hose pipe in the window of the car and me not reporting him missing to the police?" Obviously I didn't want that so I made the report but then questions are asked about whether there is anything that you know, and then you have to give a bit more, so that was that.

The police came round to collect pictures and take details and then, out of nowhere, at about half past four in the morning, just as the police were there, his car pulls in the drive. The police went and in he came; he was in a dreadful state. He'd obviously been drinking and had been sick and was shivering uncontrollably. He was just in an absolutely terrible state. It wasn't apparent until later that he had taken lots of Paracetamol. I tried to find out what's going to happen next, where we're at, what has gone on but he wasn't really in a fit state to have a conversation, so I put him to bed. I think I stayed up all night but in the morning he was up and out, showered and ready by half past eight to go out again.

When he came back, I had to go through things and matters were obviously going to follow an inevitable path. He became more forthcoming about some of the things that had gone on.

I hadn't let Beth know what had gone on until I had an idea in my head about what had gone on and what was going to happen next. She didn't have to know at that point: she had her driving test and her end-of-term ball. She looked marvellous in her outfit and went off and had an absolutely fantastic time. I wanted her to stay oblivious to it all for as long as she possibly could. I think she went home to her mother's that weekend, so that was her out of the way and it was just us and the two little ones. We did what we would normally have done with the kids and, you know, saw this friend or that friend.

I really can't remember the sequence of days as I was still on this kind of automatic pilot. He had commitments, which was absurd really, but anyway he had to do it. That weekend was when … it was awful, really awful you know, just … he was just inconsolable, could see no future. It was … he had ruined all of our lives and he could see absolutely no, no prospect that he could be, or deserved to be, forgiven.

We got to the next week (possibly the day after the Bank Holiday Monday), and again, it was suit on, papers ready for whatever commitment he had. It hadn't been apparent when he came back that he'd taken tablets, but then we had talked about that and then we had the most ridiculous conversations about suicide, how it would be better, you know, for the kids, the kids wouldn't be tarnished or labelled or we – me and them – wouldn't be as stigmatised if, you know, if he had … ridiculous conversations about suicide. I think, actually, initially I really quite wanted him to … to do it. I didn't feel that all of the time but you have kind of episodes where you float in and out of ideas, and I did consider that that would be tidier but I am not at all proud of that.

Anyway, the next week he took himself off and again and the sort of thing happened where he wasn't contactable on the phone. This continues and then it gets to teatime and he is not where he said he's going to be and it gets to some ridiculous time of night and I reported him missing again. He was gone for two days that time and I honestly didn't think that he would come back because it was longer this time. Beth had gone to her mother's in Chester, so I had to ring June [Beth's and Matthew's mother] and explain exactly what had happened, what I knew. His dad was contacted. Obviously, Tom's office then had to know.

It was awful, it was really, really dreadful, and I really honestly didn't hold out any hope that he would come back at all. His phone accepted messages and the world and his wife rang and left messages and it was … Beth and Matt came up just to see if they could do anything. I said, "It's probably better if you go down back home", so they went back home. It was just … it was awful, it was really, really awful; it was the most indescribably awful time. He came back, you know, just … a phone call, a brief phone call two days later on a teatime, early evening: the phone went and it was him. I said, "Where are you?", and I said "Just come home! Whatever has happened, just come home!" He turned up and he was desperately poorly. He had spent two days drinking God knows how much spirits, taken God knows how many Paracetamol. I rang a friend, got her to come round to look after the kids. I bathed the kids and put them to bed and I said, "I'll have to take you down to the hospital."

I got him changed, put him in the car with a bucket (in case he was going to be sick) and a drink of water. Again, he wasn't in a fit state to have a conversation, but it went along the lines of, "Is this because there are things you haven't told me and because you know some of the things … That it's true, what's being said is true?" And, yes, he just sat and said some things that were just absolutely dreadful and just how sorry he was and that was it. We got to the hospital – that was the most pressing thing. He was hospitalised, spent, I think, two or three days on a ward in the general hospital and was then transferred to a psychiatric hospital and then moved to the psychiatric ward of the hospital near where we were and he was there for weeks until he was ... until his arrest – he was actually arrested in the hospital.

From my experience, I don't think that people, whatever the hole they're in, whatever they've done – that people tend to tell you the truth in one kind of nice, tidy, organised lump; you tend to get instalments and people try and pave the way. So, I think that that's what I'd had, in terms of the talk of access to pornography on the internet, which again was a shock, and in terms of involvement and participation in chatrooms. So, it was kind of drips really, but you had to, kind of, rethink because there was obviously more in the gaps than what was laid out in front of you and it was impossible not to think that. But I do think that from that point onwards he was honest about what he had done and I think, basically, there wasn't anything else to be. Despite the fact that he'd come back, I think that he thought that everything was lost anyway. I don't think he had the slightest notion in his head that I would stick by him or the family would or that, you know, he was worthy of any forgiveness. I don't think he had that idea at all, even as the vaguest possibility.

I didn't have any great experience of dealing with computers because mostly then [when I was working] they weren't on the go. I didn't know anything about the degrees of this kind of thing, the kind of categories of severity [of child pornography]; didn't know anything about that at all. I didn't have any kind of official version of what it was he had seen but just from what he had said, I knew that among whatever it was he had looked at, he'd made reference to some pictures of, I don't know, whether. ... children being tortured and abused among whatever this mass was. The first kind of indication about numbers [of images] was weeks later at the [child protection] case conference – obviously my children were subject to a case conference – and that was really the first clue about numbers.

There wasn't really a great deal of let-up from being stunned. It was inconceivable. I don't really know if I knew what to think or ... Why would he do that? This was not him or anybody else, not any kind of right-thinking person. Why would anybody choose this course of action? Why would he wish to access pornography on the computer and anything else? Beyond that it is even more dumbfounding. I suppose the next thing was the numbers, because the numbers went into thousands and, you know, you think again: how ... when could all of this have been done? He spent hours and hours and hours working in the study often on the computer and that was obviously time when that is what he was doing.

I didn't have the vaguest idea, had no idea. Our study was downstairs and if you walked in the door you wouldn't be able to see the computer screen. If you walked in with a cup of coffee all you were presented with was somebody behind the desk, facing the door.

Our routine would be that he would come home on an evening, and it was always dinner with Mark and Beth because Sarah was too small, and then time with Mark before we bathed him and put him to bed and then we would have a little bit of time before he would start work, so his work or preparation was about half past nine – ten o'clock onwards. We would sit and … I mean, you think … you have to scrutinise everything … was that really. … did I have a … was I being realistic … was that really how it happened? But for him to have progressed as far as he did in such a short period of time, he had to sit and really work, because when you start you don't just get one or two cases, you get absolutely piles and piles, you know, a pile this high of separate case papers which you have to prepare initially for the magistrate's court. He would never ever fail to prepare them. People would ring him up for advice, not just written, formal advice but advice and guidance for other things and he would never not do it. It was a massively high level of pressure, so undoubtedly in amongst the time that I'd supposed he was just doing work and preparing what he had to prepare, that was really the only time he could have done it. Family life involved being up really early in the morning and him being out of the house by eight o'clock and weekends were our time so, in amongst the sitting in the study, in the wee small hours there was all this as well.

He had a chance to see the children. I took them to hospital to see him because that was very, very important for Mark. It was very, very important to keep Tom alive and he was in an absolutely dreadful state in hospital. The children were with me, and you have to revisit everything; you revisit how things were with my stepchildren, when they were small. Had I ever seen anything that I was unhappy with? Had he ever said anything that was inappropriate? Had any concerns ever arisen? And the answer to that was a resounding "No!" You have to trawl backwards and forwards through that with Mark and Sarah: had there ever been anything at all that would have suggested any sexual interest in the children, anything inappropriate, and there wasn't. But then, you think, "Well, am I just saying that?" I have always been very actively involved in everything, in the time that we have spent with my stepchildren when they were small, and I have been around all the time for my children and there wasn't anything … there's nothing that I'd seen or heard. Anybody's children that we had ever been in contact with – had he ever said anything that was concerning and I did have to go through all this, I mean, I do think that I'm very aware. But then I'd think, "Are you just saying this out of convenience for yourself? Are you just saying this because it's what you want to believe?" You don't want there to be any triggering but, you know, the bottom line is I was confident in myself as a parent and I was confident in our sort of family life together. When Matt and Beth came up, when he was in hospital for those weeks, I asked them. It wasn't something that I wanted to have to say but it had to, you have to. Even though it's not what you want to do, that's exactly what you have to do: you have to explore things that you don't want to know about because it's no use not knowing.

Beth is now 23, so she would have been nearly 18 then and Matt would have been four years older. They were absolutely stunned, absolutely stunned. Everybody was; Tom's dad was, his brother was; everybody, his colleagues, just everybody, just incredulous because it was completely at odds with who he is, who you believed him to be; just stunned.

Dick, Tom's dad, was just absolutely shocked. He came up and saw me. I think he just didn't know what to do. It's a different generation and Tom's the oldest, he was always the kind of blue-eyed boy, he'd progressed further than his three brothers, and he'd climbed mighty high and had fallen from grace. Initially, Tom's dad didn't really know what he wanted to do, how he wanted to react and then he wrote him a letter, saying he was his son, he loved him and that whatever happened he would stick by him. That's not to say that it was sugary sweet but it was a fantastic letter and he did give Tom something to cling to.

But on the first visit to the hospital, he said in very blunt terms, "Well you have really fucked things up, you have really fucked your life up haven't you?" Tom also had quite quickly accepted some of that from Matt. He and Beth, they're very different. Matt plays his cards much more closely to his chest than Beth does. She can articulate, can shout and scream and cry and demonstrate her emotions. Matt is more like his dad, he finds it far more difficult to do that. Tom was going have to take some of this from Dick and from me but, obviously, it wasn't appropriate on the occasions when I visited when I had the little ones there. Beth had every right to be extremely disappointed in him and was very, very angry with him. Despite the fact that he was in this huge, black abyss and was on suicide watch, he still had to be prepared to take some of this.

After he was arrested he was charged with possessing child pornography and the case had to be taken out of this circuit and he ended up going across to Leeds. His dad went to collect him from court and then he went back to his dad's in South Yorkshire. I went across and spent weekends visiting and that's how we went on for the year until trial.

I haven't got any criticism of the police or social services per se, but I think some of the things they did were insensitive. Tom was arrested from hospital, and I think that was unnecessary and insensitive. He wasn't going to go anywhere and I would not have been complicit in allowing him to bugger off or anything like that. He was arrested at whatever time it was early in the morning, and the hospital rang me and said that it had happened. The social worker happened to be at my house and scuttled off like a scalded cat, so I think that there was something … well, that detail doesn't matter now. It was in the press very quickly after that and that kind of compelled me to order my priorities: I had to tell Beth and that had to come from me, so that had to be done first, and I had to tell Tom's dad and sort out my family.

Beth was living with us but it was the end of term and then there was a period between exams, so she has always moved kind of up and down quite frequently between our house and her mother's, so that had to be done. Then it was just intolerable that people wouldn't hear it from me, so I went to church that weekend and asked if everybody would mind staying behind afterwards and I just explained, in very brief terms, basically what had happened and where he was and that was it and that's how I've been. I would hope that's how everybody would judge that I've been from the start.

I live in a very small town in a cul-de-sac and had been going to church and was very friendly with the minister at the time and a few people in the village and in the church. I thought that was the most honourable thing to do really and then people could make their own minds up how they wished to proceed from there. I have to say everybody has been very, very kind to me and the children. My neighbours have been fantastic.

That was then. I think that there has been some more negative reaction since Tom was released from prison. I think people have found that while it was quite easy to support me and the children, it's an altogether more difficult thing now for some people who will perceive that by wishing to rebuild family life that I'm somehow giving a sign of approval for what he's done and that's just not true whatsoever. I never have, and until I draw my last breath I will never think that what he's done was anything other than completely, absolutely and profoundly wrong. From everything that I've known about him, it's hard to set off and balance right and wrong but I don't give approval and I never ever will. If there was ever anything that concerned me in any way, to any degree, I wouldn't, I just wouldn't, I couldn't ... it would be impossible for me to endure anything like this again and I wouldn't have any hesitation in ... I just can't even go there, but you know, it's just very hard to balance: Tom is a good person who has done a very bad thing.

I am not saying that moving home is never going be, I'm not saying that that won't ever happen, but I don't believe in running away from things, and I don't think I could live a lie. What would you do? My initial thought was, "Well he's not there, you've got to sort out all of this," and then I said, "Bloody hell, I haven't worked for three years, what on earth am I going do? And there's this tiny baby: what do you do?" Your first reaction is, "Well, I'll have to sell the house," and 'laughingly' I thought that in that week it would sell and it didn't so then you think, "Well, I can't just sit around doing nothing, I have to find some work. What can I do?", so it was a bit like that. The decisions that had to be made were so kind of enormous you just can't just think.

Where was I going to move to? I can't say I didn't explore possibilities of where I could move to: where will people not know you? But then you isolate yourself and then what do you do? How do you conduct yourself? You make friends with somebody: what do you choose to tell them and not tell them? Then you get to know somebody and you build up a relationship with them, and you either don't tell them, in which case is it genuine, or you do tell them and then you are possibly in the same situation that you were? So what do you do? Do you keep on running? That's not the sort of life that I want for the children and it really wasn't the sort of example that I wanted to set for Matt or Beth. They are adults, but often there are adult bodies but sometimes there's something inside of them that's definitely rendered vulnerable and helpless and childlike by these circumstances and that's not the sort of example that you can be. That responsibility was probably the greatest driver – that, plus keeping him alive.

I didn't really think that it was a sensible thing to do, to rush in and make these momentous decisions about where you were going to be and how you were going to do; it just wasn't practical. I had to start paying the bills, that had to be done straight away, or at least make some inroads into that and sort things out financially somehow, that had to be done. But I think, generally, running … I mean it's … I think you have to kind of rely on the values that you've been brought up with and what your sense of right and wrong is, your sense of duty and obligation, and running away and not taking responsibility was just not an option.

[*Were your religious beliefs important to you at this time?*] Massively, absolutely massively. As a child you went to Sunday school and so I was brought up with choir and Brownies and Sunday school. But when you're stuck, when you're really, really stuck … I think, as well as losing my parents, the previous two years, having the difficulties that we'd had, it was very, very important. It doesn't always guard you against thinking completely the wrong things, but it's been massively important … you know, day and night when you can't sleep …

[*Do you do pray?*] All the time, all the time. When I've lain awake and been absolutely terrified, you know, about how to steer this, how to endure this, how to steer the situation, how to get everybody through, to make the right decisions for the right reasons. So, yes, I pray, just for everything, just for the strength to get up and get out of bed in the morning. Mark and Sarah are really, really proud of us. I suppose time will tell. I won't even hope to be sitting around in 10 or 15 years' time for them to say that they have had a happy, well-balanced childhood. How they turn out will be the test of it all, but I think and I hope that they are probably about as unaffected as you can get.

Mark has had to be told more things than his sister because again there's little things happened whereby there have been risks that other people might say things and I won't have that. They will be told the truth, but it will be by me. I'm really, really proud of the fact that I've got them to this point and Matt and Beth, as well, and everybody's sane and happy. I was determined that they wouldn't have their memory of their mother being a basket case or in bits, and them not having a good time, plodding in wellies, sitting drawing things, picking blackberries, and just doing nice things. But it was very, very hard where there was the period of time when they had to get used – or Mark especially – had to get used to daddy not being around all the time. Then daddy was living at Gran's flat. daddy was in hospital and daddy was at Granddad's. So all of a sudden, especially for him, daddy just wasn't around any more and he only got to speak to him a couple of times a week on the phone and why was that? But, you know, he was fantastic.

I explained it by being very careful about how much information he was given, if I could fob it off for a while or distract him, but there were times when you can't do that very much longer. I had to tell Mark that his daddy was in prison because there was a slight possibility (and it didn't happen) that through school somebody might have said something and I couldn't risk that. The mechanics of it haven't yet been explained, I didn't think that was age appropriate.

Mark saw his dad in hospital and knew that that he wasn't very well, that he wasn't very well in his head. I've explained that daddy has done something very, very wrong and he was arrested by the police, and the courts said he had to go to prison. That's very important to me. Mark has got a very strong sense of right and wrong and if people do things that are unkind or unfair, it's important that that's not sort of swayed, that the right and wrong that applied to me and him also applied to daddy. I feel that I've borne the sort of hardship of the decisions that Tom created by his behaviour and, as a consequence, by the legal system by its usual process. I think I've probably had to bear that the hardest. But you can't fault what happened. Tom did something that was very wrong and he had to be punished, the same as anyone else would have to be punished and I want Mark to know that and, in the future, to understand that.

Mark was sort of waiting for it and I remember making the decision that it is going to have to be now that we tell him. This was, you know, some time into the sentence (I think it was in the summer holidays and Tom had been sentenced in May). We were driving somewhere and he asked the question and I remember thinking, "I'm going to have to pull over and deal with it; this is an appropriate time to deal with it now." So the where he is? "In prison," and he was absolutely horrified. Obviously the "why?" question was asked. And I said that it was because he has done something very, very wrong and it was, "Well, what's he done?" I couldn't tell you the words, but it was along the lines of "that's not something for you to think about now, that's something we'll talk about when you're bigger", and then I think he was more, well, what will it be like, kind of trying to visualise the kind of routine Tom would be in, and all the rest of it and that sort of thing.

I think only once in conversation did he say on the phone to Tom: "Are you still in prison?" I don't know where he thought he would have gone! But there has only ever been one reference to Tom about that and we have had opportunities in conversation arise where you can link things, you know about people making wrong decisions, how you have got to think of consequences and things like that.

I think he's very confident, I think [Mark and Sarah] are both very confident but they're both very, very confident in me and I think they will ask things when they want to know and I won't avoid having a conversation. We will have to have conversations as incidents occur, as things are mentioned, perhaps as things are said, as things have to be explained, but they're very, very lucky because we've got a fantastic … I've got a fantastic relationship with them both, and they do talk very freely. Tom does worry about them and he does feel things very deeply and he doesn't bottle things up and I think they're fortunate again in that, and especially with both Beth and Matt, but especially with Beth because she's been around for much of Mark's little life. He's got a great ally and another sounding board in his big sister.

I think, as you look back on things, there was a period when – it wasn't walking into the study and finding him switching off the computer or something like that – there were lots of things, like I did know that he was extremely stressed. But, then, given the kind of rapid sequence of events that had happened before, that was entirely understandable, given how hard he was working and the long hours, the financial pressure, the fact that I wasn't well. But there was definitely something: he hadn't drunk for years and he was drinking and sort of not being honest about it. He looked dreadful, he looked unwell; I wouldn't have been surprised if he'd had a nervous breakdown. I wouldn't have been surprised if he somehow crumbled because of everything that had gone on before, but this was just not at all what I had expected to happen.

I wanted us to be a family again and I think that I had it in my head from quite early on. I don't think you know how you're going to feel about things until it's upon you really. I suppose I was confident in what I was doing when I was visiting him in hospital, I was confident in what I was doing when I was visiting at weekends when he was at his father's home. I suppose the term of imprisonment, when I was completely on my own, would have given me the break or a great period of thinking time.

It's just what, what do you believe about this person? Do you believe they have done this awful thing? Absolutely, yes! Do you believe that you've missed something in the past, and I don't think that I have. Had things gone on with Matt or Beth or anybody else? Has there been any sign of this behaviour in the past and have I missed it somehow? I don't think that's the case. Nobody that I've spoken to that's known Tom for any great length of time thinks that's the case either.

I could have walked away, I could still walk away. Do I think that's the right thing to do and I do I think that's the right thing to do for me? Do I think that's the right thing to do for him? This is not in order of priority, but do I think it's the right thing for Mark and Sarah? I don't think it's the right thing to do for Mark and Sarah, I don't think it's the right thing for Matt and Beth. I don't think it's the right thing for his dad. But if I didn't feel as confident about the past, if I had any kind of unanswered questions, then I don't think I would feel like this. If Tom had laid hands on Matt, Beth, Mark or Sarah I wouldn't feel like this and I wouldn't be making this decision and if there were ever any repeat or any suggestion of repetition of any of this sort of behaviour then I wouldn't be sticking around.

He'd done an SOTP [Sexual Offender Treatment Programme] course in prison and he made himself available for everything that was on offer and, again, had he not done that, that would have been another factor in my decision-making process.

I am very aware of how sensitive the situation is and how it affects your behaviour and how it affects how you do things and how it affects how we do things as a family. I can't see there ever being circumstances where, for example, Tom would be able to go and pick the kids up from school – that will never happen – or attend the Christmas performances. We have to be very careful.

I would never wittingly put Mark or Sarah in the position where anything you know ... we do go out together as a family, but we have to be very considered about how we do that. It will leave a legacy for ever but I don't think that that difficulty necessarily means it's impossible. I think that if you are sensible and prepared and you get advice and guidance from all possible sources, I don't think that that difficulty does mean things are impossible. I do think that things we do ... well, perhaps you just have to find a different way of doing them.

Thank God! I'm sensible. I do think that's one of my biggest assets, being sensible and being practical. I think that if you have that and you believe that something's right, then you don't put blinkers on and you don't abandon the possibility of getting more information or having to take on board other things. I think if you do believe a thing's all right then that's the course you have to steer, really.

Cheryl Eliot

"I'm suffering for what he's done. It's the price you have to pay"

Cheryl Eliot is 36 and has lived with Graham Byers for six and a half years. She has an 18-year-old son, Michael, who lives with her and Graham, and a 15-year-old son, Jamie, and a daughter, Trudi, aged 8, by a previous marriage. Trudi, like Jamie, lives with her father. She and Graham have a 3-year-old son, Gus. (Graham has a daughter, Kim, aged 17, with whom he now has no contact.) Cheryl was abused by her father, with whom, "believe it or not", she is still in contact. Her first husband was physically violent toward her. Her son, Jamie, had been abused by her half-brother and her cousin, during which time she says Graham was "a rock". The shock was all the greater, then, when she discovered that Graham had kept from her a conviction for the abuse of a 7-year-old girl some years before they met. In 2007 it emerged that he had, in fact, abused another girl of about the same age. Now 21, she had gone to the police and it turned out, coincidentally, that she was a friend of Cheryl's sister and Cheryl had also known her. Graham confessed immediately to the offence and received a two-year suspended sentence. Having hardly recovered from the shock of his first deception, the news of his other offence severely jolted Cheryl's faith in his trustworthiness. Yet she has resisted all pressure by social workers to separate from him. Graham refers to their relationship as a "success story"; it was one of the reasons why he agreed to be interviewed. Cheryl is more sceptical about the progress they have made. He tells his story on page 117.

We've been together just about six and a half years now. We met through my auntie's husband. He was working with Graham at the time and he thought it was a good idea that we got together because he knew Graham was single and he knew I was single as well.

About a year into the relationship, Graham started acting a bit peculiar and he came to me house one day – he wasn't living with me then, but he was seeing me – and just said the social workers were coming to see me and told me that he was on the sex offenders' register because he had abused a little girl. I think it was about '97 when this had actually happened, so it was a long time ago.

I was fuming at first because previous to that, it happened in me family and Graham had been like a rock to me and he could have told me then, but he didn't. I had made one comment and I'd said, "Oh, even if he has done it he's not gonna admit to it," and Graham said, "Why?" and I said, "Well, would you?" and he could have said then, you know, he had the opportunity to say it and that's what annoyed me more, I think, about not telling me – he could have told me then.

[*Did you say, "Why didn't you tell me?"*] Oh yes! And a few other choice words as well, but he really told me because five minutes later they were at the door, police and social workers, and it was just … I wasn't very happy.

Me son Jamie (he was only young, maybe 7 or 8) had been abused by me half-brother and his cousin as well, but he kept it all quiet, hadn't told anybody and then he had gone to school and it come out. He'd kept me in the dark as well, nobody told me, I didn't know until me mam phoned me up telling me, because social services had told her because it was her son who did it – so I was just kept in the dark all the way through.

There was abuse in [my childhood]. It was me father when I was 16, left school, I'd had a barney with me mam, so she kicked me out, and I went to live with me dad. Well, I mean, he did abuse me but he didn't, like, penetrate or anything like that. It just happened the once and then I moved out. Strange as it may sound I do, yes, have contact with him.

Yeah, [my mother knew about this], she didn't straight away, 'cos I went to live up in Scotland and she came up there to drag me back, 'cos I'd gone with … who I ended up marrying, so she come to drag me back and I told her what had happened. It was all hushed up, I don't know … I don't think they believed me, to tell you the truth.

It was awful [to learn about Graham] because I have always ever hated men that do that. You know, you do anyway, but when it's happened to you it's like more … even worse and Graham knew about the abuse off me dad as well.

[*Did you think, what is it about me, why am I attracting people like this?*] Yeah, I did yeah. I don't so much now, but I did before I had this [Parents for Protection] course here [at Mosaic] yeah, because I'd had … I did have an abusive relationship with someone who I married as well. He never sexually abused me but he used to hit me and me confidence was right low so, some people think that's why I've stayed with Graham because I've got no confidence. But I do, because I changed after I got the guts to finish my relationship with me first husband and then I just changed into a different person and I will never let anyone hurt me again. I did.

I described Graham as me knight in shining armour. When I met him he was just too good to be true, which is usually the case, it's usually right, isn't it, if you see it?

I think at first I … deep down … I don't think I believed he'd done it at first, because he said he hadn't to me and I think I probably believed him, but there was always the doubt there niggling, you know, at the back of my mind but I don't know … I had finally found this lovely man who loved me and he was lovely to me and treated me good.

He's told me [about the other abuses] and I've learnt through this course here, and then going on this course has learnt him to be a lot more open. I did learn about what he had done because of social services and I had to know through solicitors and everything so, like I say, it's just confusing remembering because he did get accused of the first ... well, he got – what's the word? I can't think of the word – like the first one, he did get caught for it and punished. The second girl was actually not too long ago, she was, like, what they call an historic one. She is about 21 now so she had just come forward last year. They did both happen around the same time, but she didn't come forward then so, now he is on the sex offenders' register again because he didn't admit to it all them years ago.

She came forward at the beginning of last year and he hadn't told me. I was fuming again, very, very ... especially because as I thought we had made a breakthrough, like, with me doing this course, 'cos I was having a hard time when I came to do this and I got to the end of the course and I did finally realise he had done it. I needed to go home and confront him which I did do eventually and he broke down. He was upfront with me and I just felt like a weight had been lifted. I thought, "Oh great, we can communicate about it now," and then that happened and again he was very cagey about it, didn't tell me the police had been 'cos I was at work when they'd came and he lied, yes. I said, "What's it about?" He said, "I don't know" but he must have known fine well what it was about and who it was. That's the most annoying thing about him that he just doesn't tell me, he thinks by hiding it, it's gonna go away and it's not. It makes you wonder if there is gonna be any more crawling out the woodwork in years to come. I don't know, it happened once, I've asked him, and he said no but he's said no before.

Oh well, when it happened again last year, I just ... I was really ready for ending it, I just couldn't cope with it any more and, to be honest with you, I know you say you shouldn't stay together for your children because I've tried it before meself and I know it doesn't work, but I think that was the main reason at that time and while now we are getting over it, we're still not there, we're not as successful as he claims we are.

He says he sees what I've gone through and understands but I don't think he does and I've never, ever lost me rag with him or been horrible about it either but I did a few weeks ago, I chucked it back in his face, type of thing. It's the first time I've ever done it, but it just needs to be said sometimes.

I mean, to be honest, I didn't really feel that bad [about Gus] because I know that he's not been proven to be a risk to boys because of he did a thing at the SBU [Sexual Abuse Unit] a few years ago and me little girl's not with us anyway. Graham's not allowed any contact with her, so she can come over and sleep and stay for tea, but Graham has to go out of the house, so he sleeps in the car, so he never sees Trudi anyway, so that wasn't what was worrying me. He's not allowed to see her at all, no contact, hopefully that might change after this ... you know after he's finished this course [the relapse prevention course] he can do a bit more with Trudi.

We had to tell her [why this is] when she was like really little, which annoyed me because I didn't think she should have to know but the social worker said, yes she should, but at least she knows the real reason why: it's not 'cos the social worker's saying, "'cos it's your mam doesn't want you any more" and all that. She's had a bad time with them, so at least she knows it isn't because of that and she knows what the real reason is.

Jamie and Trudi come over and, like, Graham's not allowed any contact with Jamie because he's been abused so they think he might be, like, vulnerable, but I mean as he's getting older obviously it's improving and that. Michael's fine (he's the 18-year-old). I mean, he obviously wasn't happy when he found out. He was okay the first time around because I think he was a bit like me, he didn't believe Graham had done it, you know, but after this second one I think … I dunno he's a funny one, very independent 'cos we had to fight to get him back with us. He wanted to come home so he had to go in front of the judge and say, like, why he wanted to come back and show that he did understand what Graham had done. But I think he does like Graham and he gets on all right with him, not brilliantly 'cos he's, like, it's stepson–stepdad scenario but they get on all right. I think Michael maybe tolerates him because I like him so much and I want him to be there so, just so long as me mam's happy, he'd say. He doesn't really talk about it a great deal.

Trudi, she's all right, I mean, like I say, she understands. We had a bit of a bad time 'cos she thought I loved Graham more than I love her and I've had to try and explain that that isn't really the case and things just happen and then when I went on to have my son with Graham and he's allowed to be at home as well … but she is getting better and she isn't too bad now.

I think they should know because I know Gus's gonna love his dad no matter what you do, but I don't know. I don't think Graham will be happy about him knowing, but me kids have had to know, that's what annoys us 'cos Graham's got a daughter to a previous marriage as well and she doesn't know. She'll be 17 now; he doesn't really see her because we don't know where she lives. We tried to get in contact with her, we send her birthday cards through the grandparents, but she's never been back in touch. I do sometimes [think I know why that is] because his ex-wife was … I dunno, not nice, she had her moments, one minute she was fine with us, the next …

[*Has it passed through your mind that he had abused his daughter?*] That she might know about her dad? No, that's not … no, because I've seen him with Kim. Even, when I did this course, I expressed that to them, they said it's actually a good thing that he didn't 'cos he gets very upset if you talk about Kim in that way and they did believe that he hasn't, like, thingied Kim. And I think hearing it from someone that who's, like, professional as well … I'm not saying that they're right – he could have – but I think he sees that [abusing his own daughter] as totally wrong. I know it might sound a bit hypocritical but you know …

I fell out with my family, started talking to them again and fell out again at the moment when it all happened again. It wasn't too bad, I mean obviously people were upset and they came round slowly to actually come into the house again but after last year I didn't talk to me mam for, oh, about eight months I think, just because I didn't want to face her. She didn't get into contact with me either so I fell out with them.

I didn't fall out with my sister so much, but I didn't contact her either because it was her friend that had come forward, like the historic one. It turned out that she had been at school with her so she knows her and, I mean, I even know her so that was quite an annoying time. Graham didn't know I'd known her – I knew her when she was about 15 – but then, like, me granda took ill I'd heard off my dad, so I just texted me mam and just started talking and everything's been all right from there. At first I didn't mention Graham's name if I was talking to her but now it's not too bad and she will pop to the house now and again. I wouldn't say she's brilliant with him but I think she's a bit more understanding now.

We don't talk about it [staying with Graham] though. When I made it up with me mam, when I phoned up when my granda was bad and I said something – I didn't know if she'd want me to phone. I didn't know, she might have slammed the phone down, but she said, "Oh, you know what are we like," and that's it, you know, we fall out and then we just start talking again, but we never go over why we fell out in the first place.

I talk to my dad about it but he … as strange as that sounds, he's quite glad I told him, but he's annoying as well, 'cos he's never admitted to what he's done to me so if I see him frowning upon what Graham's done, that annoys me. No, I've never confronted him about it. I did at the time, straight away but years and years and years have gone by and social services found out about it, so he wasn't allowed to have contact with Trudi and he actually blamed me for that. "Oh, okay then it's nothing to do with what you did then, dad." So I fall out with me dad now and again as well.

A couple of close people that I've worked with when it all came out though, they know and we did have one in the street that did know. I thought that she was a friend and the fella that she was with. We ended up getting a load of hassle off him, he was smashing me windows, so I just don't tell people now, which is a bit, I dunno … Graham doesn't understand this about me. I've never spoke about it to him but people at work if they like me, I feel like a fraud 'cos they're not liking the real me because I'm with a sex offender and what would they think? But some people you do want to tell. What would they think if they knew that? They probably wouldn't like me then, but you can't … you just can't tell people no matter how good a friend you think they are, you just … I've often nearly told somebody and then the next day think, "Oh, I'm that pleased I didn't," you know.

He got back on the offenders register and got a suspended sentence for two years [for the most recent offence], so if anything else happens in that two years he could end up in prison, but he did actually get commended for pleading guilty, 'cos he done it straight away when he went to the police station. He just said, "Yes, I've done it," and he held his hands up so, which is a good thing 'cos it spared the girl having to go to court.

Police and social workers were horrible. Not very nice, all just so judgemental. They don't get to know the real you, they just, you know, tar you with a brush and that is it – oh, with him you shouldn't be and that is it! End of story. They just don't listen to you. You know, I've been told I'm an intelligent woman but you never get that off them. It's just they don't get to know the real you, barge into your house and tell you this, this and this, and this is how it's going to be. I've had quite a bad time with them actually, lots of fights, and they didn't want me to keep Gus, our son. He was put on the [at risk] register before he was even born which my solicitor – luckily, I had a good solicitor – said, "He's [Graham's] no risk to boys". I'd had a scan showing it was gonna be a boy, I know it's not a 100 per cent but why they should put Gus on the register when he wasn't here, you know it's so ... unfair and unjust.

I had contact with teachers when Michael was at school still. They were all fine actually, really good. I was dreading seeing them but really good. Quite understanding if Michael got a bit too much leeway at school because of it, but they were really, really good about it, never looked down their noses at me; no, just really nice.

I wouldn't say reluctantly, very wary, nervous and petrified [in coming to the Partners for Protection course] 'cos me and Graham had actually been trying to get on this course – like me on one of them, him on the other one – for, oh, about two years I think before we actually got on it and nobody would fund it. They said we had to pay ourselves for it but my solicitor was fighting, saying to social services, "It's you that want them to split up, so you should fund it," and they wouldn't. In the end it was the Legal Aid, we got it through a loophole in the Legal Aid, finally got them to pay but social services have took the credit for paying for it!

I knew it would go good for us getting on it and, you know, proving that I could look after me children and protect them and I didn't know if it was true or not [about what he had done]. Hopefully, it was helping Graham if he got on one.

Before I did the course, no, I didn't know [about sex offending]. I will protect me children no matter what but I was very naive to tell you the truth. When I'd finished the course I even said at the end of it, you don't realise how naive and daft you've been. It opens your eyes because I didn't think he had done it. Well, maybe it was always there, like I say, in the back of me mind that he had done it, so I did used to watch out but I think as time had gone on I maybes would have trusted him with Trudi had they ever been allowed to be together, but now I wouldn't. But even if he passes this course with flying colours, I will not leave him [with her] and I wouldn't go to the shop even for five minutes so it just opens your eyes, coming on this really.

I mean, I'd been told about grooming and that but you just ... I don't think it sinks in properly until you actually come on the course. I mean, one of the things we actually did here was you had to act a situation out and that's when it really hit home 'cos, like, the woman doing it was pretending – obviously it had to relate to your case – so she was, like, a 7 or 8-year-old little girl pretending to be my daughter so that's when it hit home, I think, when we did that.

[*Given your own feelings are about people offending against children and your own experiences, do you feel that Graham got off lightly?*] It's a hard one, that. Mmm! I think ... I mean, it's weird 'cos obviously I'm with one [an offender] but I think it depends on the seriousness. I'm not saying none of them are serious but there's a grading to it. With Graham it was just – not "just": I know that's an awful way of putting it – just touching. I know none of it is right, it's just hard to explain, isn't it, but when it's somebody that you love you don't want them to go into prison and get killed or beat up but I think, yes, they do get off lightly. But it's not just them that suffer as well, it's the family, it's me you know, I'm suffering for what he's done, which I think is the price you have to pay, I suppose.

Life's not going to be normal. You know, my sister's got a little girl now, she doesn't come to the house when Graham's there and my son's 18 now, and he could be getting married in four years' time. What's gonna happen at the wedding, with children there? I think about the future all the time. Like me son being good at football. He got a trial for [a major league team] it was and all the time I was – I know it sounds awful – but I was hoping deep down really that he wouldn't make it because I could see the headlines, if he got picked to play for England. Graham doesn't see things like that 'cos he … I mean, he's drawing now, and he's a really good drawer. He jokes on that, "When I get noticed … " and I'm, like, "But you never can," it's just if you won the lottery, he would have to stay anonymous. Just daft little … well not, daft little things, it's things I think about every day. I don't think Graham does, he just thinks that … I mean I can't even get house insurance, believe it or not, for my contents because of Graham. If I tell them if anyone – and they always ask – has anyone got a criminal record. "Yes," I tell them. "What it is?" Oh, no, so you can't have it then, so things like that, you know, it's just normal, everyday life to anybody else.

Oh, when I told him about the insurance thing, "Of course, you can," he said and I said, "Yes, if you lie to them, if you just say, 'Oh, nobody's got a criminal record in this house,'" and suddenly your insurance is void anyway, so. I've never fronted these things about like Michael being a footballer 'cos it was a dream world at the time because he was good, but the marriage thing, like the wedding's coming up in the future. I've never talked about that to Graham, I've never brought that up.

He's quite laid back and I'm not. Now, at the moment, things are okay, not wonderful, but any relationship's hard, anyway, and then having this [news of the second conviction] added on top of it, it's just …

I wouldn't say it's mainly because of what he's done, though, to us, it's because of the way he acts sometimes and like other men does at times, you know, but I don't know if it's all linked, you know, his behavioural patterns. I worry if he does start acting up because sometimes he is quite childish – I know most men are quite childish – but he really aggravates me.

I just get scared because I don't know what he was like before when he offended so I don't know if there's … you know I don't know what his pattern was like then so, which, hopefully, I might learn when he's finished these courses, 'cos they say it's like a cycle, isn't it? There's a pattern of behaviour so if he does start to act a bit strange I do start to think, "Oh, is he gonna do that again?"

I don't think there is one specific thing, I think it's just any type of behaviour, because, as I say, I don't know what his behaviour was like when he did offend before, and it might just be me. He's just so aggravating at times, but he always puts the blame on me, it's me, it's not him, you know, and I've had that in the past as well, which is doubly annoying. No, I wouldn't say it's one specific thing that I think, "Oh no." It's not the way he acts with the children – or the child, me oldest one's not a child any more – so much and I would say it's anything specific. It's just, I get a bit panicky because, like I say, I don't know what he was like when he did offend and he gets funny moods on him and I just hope he's not gonna go back. When he's nice and normal, like I say he is a lovely fella really, most of the time.

[*Do you ever think, "I am glad I stuck with him because it helped"?*] I do, yes, like I have helped him. There was one social worker that tried giving me a lecture because I'd said I wanted to try and help him and she said, like, I shouldn't stay with him just to help him and she told me a stupid little story about a hole in the ground and he kept going back to it. She felt because I had been in a violent relationship before, I had to be one of these people and I said, "No, I'm not like that, I just do want to help Graham – he's worth helping." Everybody that meets him likes him, thinks he's a lovely fella; he is nice, he's lovely to me usually. He has his off moments, perhaps he could say the same about me, but I don't stay with him to stick two fingers up at everybody like the social services, that's not why I like stay with him – I stay with him because I love him and I think he's worth the effort.

3 Child sex offenders and what we know about them

The media stereotype of the child sex offender probably reflects a popular view – the predatory "pervert", "paedo" and even "monster". This is dangerously misleading because men who sexually abuse children are not easy to characterise. They do not fit into any social category. Their histories are different. Their public face may be (and, indeed, often is) as the respectable father and husband; helpful, loving and caring. They are members of all social classes, trades and professions, the surgeon as well as the bus driver. There may be nothing about them to arouse the least suspicion that they are a danger to children, their own or other people's. In short, they may be indistinguishable from any friend, relative, workmate or neighbour.[1]

However, the sex offender may well give a different impression to his neighbours than that he gives to his family – friendly and helpful to others outside the house, cruel and manipulative within it. But even then, children who are abused may not have a uniformly negative view of him. True, an offender may be violent and cruel to his children, but he may also be kind, loving and warm toward them. Many child victims only want the abuse to stop; they want to continue a loving relationship with the abuser.

Child sex offenders may be men who are strong, in a positive sense, but they may also be weak and ineffectual. Kind or cruel. Loving or hateful. Quiet or boisterous. Stern or warm. Assertive or meek. The contrasts are endless and point only to the difficulty of characterising men who sexually abuse children.

One thing which has bedevilled a better understanding of child sex offenders and fed the stereotype is the myth of "stranger-danger": that the offender is someone who is unknown to the child. Metaphorically or literally, he lies in wait for her. This myth is fostered by the comparatively rare cases of abduction. These cases receive such widespread publicity precisely because abduction is very dramatic, but also because it is so uncommon – although their tragic nature cannot be overstated.

The extreme improbability of molestation or abduction by a stranger is in stark contrast to the far greater likelihood that a child will be abused by someone she knows: father, stepfather, mother, brother, uncle, cousin, grandfather, family friend, neighbour, baby-sitter, teacher, clergy, or other person with whom the child has regular, informal and friendly contact. These are people who are generally trusted, and yet these are the ones far more likely to abuse.

Eighty seven per cent of child sex offenders fall into this group (ChildLine 2003). As Wyre (2004) puts it, "Monsters don't get close to children, nice men do."

An official study (Marshall 1997) showed that, in 1993, 110,000 men aged 20 and over had convictions for a sexual offence against a child, although it did not include rape. This equated to one in 150 men. However, when rape was included (in the work on the Code of Practice on Foster Care) the ratio rose to one in 140 men aged 20 and over (Department of Health 2003).[2]

A sex offender may not only ingratiate himself with a child to get close to her, but he may also ingratiate himself with a child's parents for the same purpose. These days, with the existence of police checks, the sex offenders' register, and vetting and barring procedures (imperfect as these are), there are far fewer opportunities for offenders to gain positions where they can work with children either voluntarily or professionally. However, it is not uncommon for an offender to develop a relationship with a single mother so as to gain access to the woman's children.

Types of child sex offender

There is a variety of personality factors that motivate and maintain the behaviours of offenders, and researchers (Mann *et al*. 2002) and practitioners in the UK have identified a range of factors in different degrees with different offenders. One factor is the way in which sexual interest operates. Some offenders are sexually aroused mainly by children. Others may turn to sexual thoughts of children in different situations or in different mood states. Some offenders may be obsessed with sex or use sexual outlets to cope with negative moods. For others, some kind of fetish may feed their abuse. One factor that is occasionally evident with child sex offenders is one which is more common with rapists: that is, that offenders may have sadistic motives and so be aroused by the violent aspects of sex.

There are then the attitudes to sexual abuse which offenders exhibit. Some will be very ashamed of their behaviour but will "give in to temptation" under pressure. Others may not realise that they are harming children – or at least try to convince themselves that they are not doing so. Others may believe that while sexually abusing children generally is wrong, there was something about "their victim" which made it acceptable, another example of self-delusion. A minority of abusers seem to develop the view that sexual activity (which, significantly, in their terms is not seen as abuse) with children is acceptable. This may be associated sometimes with their having convinced themselves that their own experience of abuse did them no harm.

How people relate to others is the third set of variables that has been identified. Offenders may be affected by feelings of inadequacy or they may have problems in intimate relationships with other adults. Such feelings may make some feel more comfortable with children, who are non-threatening, or may even give the offender a sense of power or feed narcissistic desires. Some offenders (again, more commonly rapists) may have a desire to offend that is fed by a deep, inchoate suspicion of others, a sense of grievance against them and the world, where they see themselves as disadvantaged by others, allied with a vengefulness.

The last important set of considerations concerns the ability (or lack of it) of offenders to manage their lives. As we have seen, there is a variety of behaviours and motivations exhibited by offenders – among them, that sexual abuse is not solely related to sex; there may be problems in managing emotions; temptations may be kept under control until other emotional factors or difficult situations arise. This is analogous to some addictive behaviours, which makes a life which is free of offending difficult to contemplate.

With these considerations in mind, we can see that it is not true that the sexual orientation of all offenders is exclusively towards children. Many child sex offenders are married or live with partners, enjoying, to all intents and purposes, an ordinary life. Some sex offenders are aroused by small children, toddlers and even babies. The abuse of a child when young may continue until the child reaches adolescence and even adulthood.

Any analysis of what causes their behaviour is usually to be found, if at all, after the abuse has taken place and they have been apprehended and perhaps received treatment. However, the small number of child sex offenders who are ever apprehended, let alone the small numbers who ever get to court and *then* receive a sentence and *then* get any treatment means that our knowledge of sexual offenders is based on a comparatively tiny proportion of the overall group.

As we have seen, child sex offenders are not a homogenous group, they do share some common characteristics. For example, they are manipulative. There are ploys and actions which require an ability to manipulate, to curry favour with a child; to get her into situations where abuse can take place; to convince her (as they do very often) that this is a game which no one else needs to know about; or that there will be adverse consequences if anyone finds out (which is not necessarily a physical threat against the child but something "kindly" meant). When discovered, an offender may express remorse. This may be genuine, but it may also be another use of these manipulative skills. It may be an attempt by the offender to lessen the anger that others feel against him, to give others some kind of assurance that his actions will not be repeated, or he may be fearful for the repercussions for himself now that others have found out.

Sexual abuse can also be analysed in terms of cycles. While Finkelhor (1984) and Wolf (1984) formulated their cycles some while ago, they remain useful in understanding the process through which many abusers go on to abuse. They also identified many of the factors described above.

Finkelhor (1984) constructed a step-by-step progress of how abuse takes place, which requires the following preconditions:

- the motivation to abuse
- overcoming internal inhibitions to abuse
- overcoming external inhibitors to abuse
- overcoming the child's possible resistance.

For each of these steps to be taken, he details a number psychological and sociological factors. For example, the psychological factors include:

- arrested emotional development; the need to feel powerful and controlling; and inadequate social skills for *motivation*;
- alcohol; impulse disorder; and a failure, within the family of an inhibition on incest in *overcoming internal inhibitors*;
- a mother who is absent or ill or is not close to the child; the social isolation of the family; a mother who is dominated or abused by the father; and a lack of supervision of the child to *overcome external inhibitors*; and
- a child who is emotionally insecure or deprived or lacks knowledge of sexual abuse; an unusual degree of trust between child and offender to *overcome the child's resistance*.

Again, to take only some of Finkelhor's factors, as he states them to obtain with regard to the sociological factors, they include:

- a masculine requirement to be dominant and powerful in a sexual relationship; the availability of child pornography; and a male tendency to sexualise emotional needs to *have the motivation to sexually abuse*;
- social tolerance of sexual interest in children; weak criminal sanctions against offenders; an inability to identify with the needs of children; and an ideology which elevates patriarchy to *overcome internal inhibitors*;
- a lack of social support; barriers to women's equality; the erosion of social networks; and a belief in the sanctity of the family to *overcome external inhibitors*; and
- the unavailability of sex education for children; and children being socially powerless to *overcome the child's resistance*.[3]

In essence, this adds up to the fact that the offender either has attitudes, specific or generalised, which give him "permission" to abuse, or he has problems of self-management which cause him to give in to temptation even if he knows it is wrong.

An offender overcomes his inhibitions about abusing by self-justification: he convinces himself of any number of things to justify his actions to himself. These include the following: that he is not hurting the child; that non-penetrative sex is not really abuse; that the child enjoys what he does; that she is to blame by, in effect, seducing him into what he did. Lack of empathy – the inability to enter into the feelings of another – is a necessary psychological defect in the abuser.

However, there is also another factor in overcoming inhibition. Not only must the offender wish to abuse but he must also psychologically prepare himself. Masturbating about deviant sexual fantasies can be used to overcome inhibitors and lead to actual abusing and then contribute to rehearsing the abuse again and so lead to further abuse. Orgasm is pleasurable and while the abuser may begin by masturbating using print or screen images of children it is but a short step *for some* offenders to seek the real object of their fantasy – the child herself. After all, the fantasy is not what the abuser *is* doing with a *pictured* or *imagined* child but what he *could* be doing with a *real* child. The offender moves from fantasy to masturbation and orgasm, stimulus and arousal. He is rehearsing what he would like to make come true. In this movement from masturbation to arousal two roles are fulfilled. The first is that it reinforces the fantasy in the person's mind and so reinforces the motivation to offend. Fantasists will often have an image of the victim liking the activity, thus reinforcing the overcoming of internal inhibitors.

This is known as the sexual arousal cycle described by Wolf (1984). It may lead to frequent offending with many or only one child or it may lead to less frequent offending with a small number of children.

If we consider a child's resistance, the obvious question is: how can children, especially perhaps more mature children, allow themselves to be abused? Why do they not draw back from the abuser in "natural" self-protection? The offender, wanting to overcome a child's resistance, is helped by the way in which most children tend to be trusting of others – unless they have been taught from an early age not to be – by the way they have been treated by others. They respond positively to offers of friendship, they respond warmly to friendliness shown to them. If someone takes an interest in them, they tend to respond positively; they may be even flattered by the interest of an adult. Most children take adults at (positive) face value and if someone appears to be a "good" person who seems to wish them no harm, they may have no reason to believe otherwise. Children do not, naturally, have much of a guard to drop. They have yet to acquire the carapace we construct in later life in relation to others.

The offender is helped by the fact that most children accept that adults know best and that they should do as they are told. A child may not even be clear as to what is happening, especially if the abuser masks it as a game. If abuse begins when the child is very young, she may become habituated to what is happening – in extreme cases, treat abuse as "normal" – and feel unable to resist as she gets older. The abuser may tell her that what happens is a secret which they share, something special to them both. He may give the child rewards of sweets, toys or other treats. He may be less strict than the child's parents, by allowing her to do things – like smoking and drinking for older children – that her parents do not allow. He may also arouse the child sexually. If a child is made to feel that she is participating, then she may find it all the harder to resist. Abusers can also threaten children into taking part – they can tell them that they will be taken into care or that if others discover what has happened, it will break up the family. In extreme cases, children may be suborned by physical violence.

When an offender fixes on a certain child he grooms her, or he grooms her parents or carers, thus gaining their trust. (Some offenders, though, do put themselves in circumstances that may or may not lead to abuse. That is, they may be alert to possibilities but without a well-thought out plan.) Grooming is a calculated act. It is the means by which the offender makes preparations so that abuse is possible. It flatters the child, makes her feel special. He creates opportunities to be with her, to gain her trust, to develop that "special relationship", to get her in a position where they are alone together, and to manipulate her into sexual activity. He may do the latter in very subtle ways. He may do it by making activities "innocent", as a game. Some young children may be too young to know that what the offender is doing is wrong. However, some abusers may lessen children's resistance by talking about sex, touch their arms and legs, or tickle them near their sexual areas. They may pretend that they are engaging in sex education. Abusers may cuddle children and act childishly so that they can be more physically close with the child. Some offenders may show children pornography.

Eldridge (1998) has formulated three different cycles: the continuous, inhibited and short-circuit cycles. The continuous cycle is one used by the offender continuously and consistently with a new victim each time. He has no internal brake on his behaviour. The inhibited cycle is when the offender may be inhibited by guilt after committing an offence or by fear of being found out. He then avoids further offending for a while but subsequently returns to the sexual arousal cycle. When he is again disinhibited the offender returns to offending with the same or a new victim. The short-circuit cycle is when an offender frequently abuses the same child. He moves from fantasy and rehearsal to sexual abuse.

The reasons for offending

What factors, then, are at work in the motivation of an offender? The offender may have low self-esteem and lack social skills, and be unable to make mature relationships with adults, although this applies to only a minority of offenders. They may have a need for power, control and attention. They may be expressing anger or need for revenge. They may seek affection and intimacy. (Affection and intimacy are basic human needs, but the offender seeks to meet these needs inappropriately.) Such traits show that, for some, abuse is not simply about sex: abusive sex can be a means to an end.

However, even if an abuser has not himself been a victim of abuse, that does not mean that some dysfunction, experience, or trauma, which is unknown, has not occurred in childhood or early adolescence has set his sexual patterns. The cultural values with which a child is raised; the models set by his father (where a father is present) and mother in their relationship; his parents' (or a parent's) attitude toward drugs, excessive alcohol and violence; his own exposure to violence, especially of a sexual kind, either in the home or, vicariously, on screen – all will influence how the child grows to view others, including, when they grow older, children.

Men who have been abused in childhood are more likely to commit abuse themselves. Again, this is not a determinist argument that gets the abuser off the hook, because many people who have been abused do *not* go on to do so themselves. The claim by an abuser that he has been abused may be used to try to excuse what he has done or to elicit sympathy. There have been indicative, rather than definitive studies of the incidence of abuse in the lives of offenders. For example, Sanderson (2004) says that 66 per cent of child sex offenders have been abused as children, but the use of lie detectors during interviews suggests that this figure may be reduced to 30 per cent. Glasser and colleagues (2001) put the percentage of male abusers who have themselves been victims at 35 per cent. Walsh (no date) says that, in his work with offenders at the Granada Institute, Ireland, he found that between 40 and 50 per cent of perpetrators were themselves abused. Only one in eight children who have been sexually abused goes on to abuse other children in adolescence (Skuse 2003).

A study which included assessing the explanations given for their crimes by 65 "child molesters", who had yet to take part in any programmes to address their offending, found that they most commonly referred to sexual gratification, the desire to alleviate a negative emotional state or a wish to experience intimacy. However, a quarter of them did not, or could not, give any explanation for what they had done (Mann and Hollin 2007).

Treatment and its effect

So far as treatment is concerned, the offender must first acknowledge that what he has done is wrong and be prepared to participate in a programme, although attendance for some offenders may be a condition of their community order. Full responsibility, and regret, will only come through treatment. (The question of offenders taking personal responsibility for their actions is a very complex area. For example, denial does not correlate statistically with risk: some people may deny because they are ashamed of what they have done (Kennington 2008).)

Does treatment work? Treatment does not imply cure. There is no "cure" for sex offending and, like the recovering alcoholic, the sex offender can relapse. But while he cannot be "cured", he can be helped to face what he has done, understand why he has done it, and what his offending patterns are. If he understands his patterns of behaviour, he can be helped to change them and to break his cycle, to manage his sexual arousal and to control his actions in future.

Questions about the efficacy of treatment are usually taken to mean whether or not reoffending rates are reduced. It is a fact, with regard to the kind of offender with whom we are dealing, that the answer to these questions must be that *good* treatment works with *some* offenders. Research indicates that well-structured programmes which are properly targeted can reduce the rate of recidivism from 17 per cent to about 10 per cent – or a reduction of 40 per cent (Hanson *et al.* 2002).

It is emphasised that treatment should always, therefore, be part of a risk management plan, as some offenders may be predisposed to reoffend for a long time. Sanderson (2004) says that between a third and a half of child sex offenders can be taught to manage their sexual arousal by children and not to act on it. Stuart and Baines (2004) refer to international research which suggests that "well-designed and delivered cognitive behavioural therapy for sex offenders reduces reconvictions by some 40 per cent". However, while Salter (2003) puts the figure at two-thirds, she also says that a third do not wish to change and will reoffend if in a position to do so (that is, when they are living back in the community).

Good treatment usually takes place in groups and is based on cognitive behavioural therapy. Such therapy helps group members to understand the feelings and behaviours which led to their offending and then to learn and rehearse strategies and skills to manage their behaviour in future.

The treatment needs to address all those factors which Mann and Hollin (2007) have identified. This is to help them manage their sexual interest; to change attitudes which allow them "excuse" their offending; to help them to manage difficulties in relationships without turning to children for emotional and sexual gratification; and to help them to manage difficulties in their lives such as emotional regulation, problem solving and impulsivity.

The methods used are important and there is little to suggest that therapies offering the offender an insight into their behaviour alone will have much effect. Methods which help offenders themselves to analyse their problems – the so-called "motivational interviewing" or "Socratic questioning" – combined with exercises, like role play, which teach new skills are important.

Critical to good treatment is the suitability of the therapeutic environment. Therapists share the feelings of almost anyone else about sex offending, yet it is their responsibility not to vent anger or disgust as many of us would do, but to channel their feelings to positive use. Marshall *et al.* (1999) have identified what they call the "cardinal virtues" of the therapist: warmth, empathy, "rewardingness" (that is, the ability to reinforce positive statements and behaviours on behalf of the offender) and directness, which is the ability to take someone through what may be a difficult process. Walsh (no date) cites "very strong evidence that there is a positive correlation between the client's perception of the quality of the therapeutic relationship and a positive outcome".

Briggs and colleagues (1998) have suggested that there should be an appropriate balance between "support and challenge" within the group. Beech, Fisher, Beckett and Scott-Fordham (1998) name "group cohesion" as an important component, while Walsh (no date) says it is "a curative factor". Beech and colleagues (2001) and Marshall *et al.* (1999) have found that punitive and confrontational regimes can actually make offenders worse in relation to key variables such as empathy with victims (Kennington 2008).

Medical treatments for offenders have been found to have limited effect, as have drug treatments. Surgery, including castration and brain surgery, has been shown to have a direct effect on the libido but can also cause permanent damage. In the long term, such treatment has led to offenders taking their own life or committing violent crime.

Medical treatment does not meet the needs of most sex offenders because it cannot deal with the non-sexual aspects of their behaviour. Discovery of the shortcomings of medical interventions was followed by a period in which, it was believed, "nothing worked", but this is now discounted in favour of comparatively new forms of treatment. It is now generally accepted, on the basis of a review of the outcomes of different kinds of treatment, that comprehensive cognitive behavioural programmes are most likely to be efficacious.

Medication has been found to be a useful complement to behavioural therapy programmes for a small number of sex offenders. Two types are sometimes used. The first is that which is "anti-libidinal", which can to help reduce the sex drive of offenders who may be hyper-aroused, while offering the opportunity for them to benefit from therapy. There are some offenders who have compulsive thoughts which they find difficult to suppress. For them the second type of medication – anti-depressants: selective serotonin reuptake inhibitors – are used.

As with all medication, there can be side effects and questions about the offender's cooperation in taking them. The effects of these drugs do not continue after the patient ceases to use them and they also do not affect some of the motivational aspects of offending in the long term (Kennington 2008).

Thus, as Marshall *et al.* (2003) point out, treatments have evolved, over three decades, from simple programmes intended to modify the behaviour of deviant sexual interest to complex and comprehensive programmes that address a broad range of issues.

The Prison Service is the largest provider of treatment programmes, which are based on cognitive behavioural therapy. It has developed the Sex Offender Treatment Programme (SOTP). Started in prisons in 1991, it is also used outside of prisons and is now the largest treatment programme of its kind in the world. Prior to SOTP there were (and are) programmes in the community run by the probation service; current community-based programmes are separate from but complementary to the prison SOTP. Indeed, all probation services in England and Wales now run accredited sex offender programmes, and they are also increasingly common in Scotland and Northern Ireland.

SOTP is believed to be most effective with high-risk and medium-risk offenders. The programme is available only to prisoners who volunteer, which they may do from a mixture of motives – a genuine desire to seek help but also the belief that attending will count as "points" in their favour with the prison authorities and the Parole Board.

The aim of SOTP is that participants should develop the skills and appropriate attitudes to lead a personally satisfying life that does not involve reoffending. This requires a greater ability on their part to empathise with victims, to be more trusting of others, to be able to better cope with personal problems and to have a clearer idea of how to achieve healthy intimacy, including sexual intimacy.

One outcome of treatment is for the offender to accept, even when treatment is complete, that he is not "cured", that he knows he may reoffend and that it is his responsibility, seeking help from others where needs be, to monitor and control his behaviour. His treatment programme should have increased his self-awareness of himself and of the way abuse works, to the extent that he will be able to watch out for, and guard against triggers to setting off such behaviour again.

In relapse prevention programmes the steps that an offender needs to take in order to control the distorted thinking that causes him to return to his former behaviour are described. He will be helped to identify high-risk factors and how to deal with them. He will be shown that he needs to stay away from situations which pose a high risk of his reoffending.

Evaluations by the Home Office have looked specifically at the effect of the SOTP on child sex offenders' readiness to admit to their behaviour; at the attitudes that encouraged offending (for example, thinking about sex with children); their social competence; and their knowledge of how to avoid relapse. Seventy-seven men were studied. It was found that the SOTP increased the level of offenders' admitting to their offence. There was a reduction in those attitudes which encouraged offending, and offenders were less likely to deny that sexual abuse had an impact on victims. Levels of social competence increased. It was considered that there had been significant changes for a third of the men (67 per cent). The longer the treatment, the better were the results maintained after release (160-hour programmes were compared with 80-hour ones). This was especially the case for highly deviant offenders (Beech *et al.* 1998).

However, there are some practical drawbacks to the effectiveness of treatment. First, some offenders do not receive sentences that are long enough for them to be treated and, of course, it makes sense to start treating those who can be treated. With regard to treatment in prison, the Criminal Justice Act 2003, with its provision for longer sentences for dangerous, violent and sexual offenders, may give greater protection to the public and allow sufficient time for treatment to take place. In 2002, there were 5,600 sex offenders in prison, yet only 839 completed the treatment that year – 111 fewer than the 950 planned by the government (Silverman and Wilson 2002). Second, even for those who do receive treatment, there is no help after release. Third, relapse programmes (which assist men not to reoffend) must come to an end (unless open-ended programmes are available) and it is then up to the offender and family members to help him to maintain his non-offending behaviour. For example, the programme run by the Northumbria Probation area allows men to attend long term if there is a need. Kennington (2008) says that this is not always taken up, and it is correct to say that treatment places tend to be allocated on the basis of completions, not necessarily of clinical need. It has been argued that not all people need to be in treatment for ever, although some may benefit from some kind of system which they believe to be supervision (for example, a meeting once a year).

Fourth (and related to the last point), the effectiveness of treatment is judged on the basis of reoffending rates. However, we must take into account low rates of detection and low conviction rates. So, where there is a conviction, it is still possible for someone to reoffend and not be discovered. As with all crime, recidivism rates are based on those who offend but who are apprehended. There is no way of knowing, with any type of crime, the numbers of offenders who reoffend but are not detected.

A very serious gap in provision is that, since the closing of the Wolvercote Clinic in 2002, in neither Great Britain nor Ireland are there any residential assessment and treatment facilities for child sex offenders. Attempts to relocate the clinic, with money allocated by government, have been frustrated by local media outbursts and public protests. This is despite the fact that research has showed the effectiveness of these programmes (Ford and Beech 2004a; Ford and Beech 2004b; Home Office *et al.* 2002).

Moreover, treatment has never been given a high priority. As Stuart and Baines (2004) note:

> There remain serious deficiencies in the number of places on appropriate treatment programmes for convicted sex offenders and a strategy to respond to this lack was seriously needed. While the structures, consistency and research base in prison and probation programmes were commendable achievements by any international comparisons, too many released sex offenders have received no treatment programme to reduce their risk prior to release. The number of community-based sex offender programmes run by the National Probation Service has risen recently to some 1,800 places per year. But as many as two-thirds of supervised sex offenders do not have access to a programme relevant to their needs because of insufficient places, inadequate length of supervision, issues of denial and suchlike. (pp. 5–6)

Prison may, at least, take offenders out of circulation and offer some of them appropriate treatment. However, the isolation behind prison walls can mirror that which some offenders may experience within the community. They will be separated from other prisoners because of the possibility that they may be attacked. This means that their company inside prison is that of other sex offenders, which may serve only to fuel their fantasies.

Other means of help

Circles of Support and Accountability work with sex offenders to help them to manage their behaviour and to avoid reoffending. The idea originated in a Mennonite community in Hamilton in Canada in 1994 and was imported to England by the Quakers.

When still in custody, an offender who is identified as being at high risk of reoffending is matched with a "circle" of about six volunteers in the area in which he will live. He becomes the "core member".

The circle, which has the support of professionals when needed, meets weekly. Most of the rest of the time the offender will be in touch with individual circle members, and contacts can range from phone calls to shopping trips or meeting for lunch. Members can help core members to try to find work and housing, as well as help if the core member starts to have inappropriate feelings or thoughts. On such occasions support may become more intensive and the offender may be challenged. Evidence both from Canada (Wilson, Picheca, and Prinzo 2007) and the UK (Bates, Saunders and Wilson 2007) suggests that circles are successful in reducing reoffending.

The Canadian research matched a group of 60 high-risk sexual offenders involved in circles with a group of 60 high-risk sexual offenders who had no such involvement after release. Those who participated in a circle had "significantly" lower rates of any type of reoffending than did their fellows. For the participants there was a 70 per cent reduction in sexual reoffending in contrast to the other group; a 57 per cent reduction in all types of violent reoffending (including that of a sexual nature: 15 per cent against 35 per cent); and an overall reduction of 35 per cent in all types of recidivism (including that which was violent and sexual: 28.3 per cent against 43.4 per cent). Moreover, when core members did reoffend, their sexual offences were "categorically less severe" than offences committed previously.

Stop It Now!, founded in 2002, seeks to intervene *before* abuse takes place. Run under the aegis of the charitable Lucy Faithfull Foundation but funded largely by government, it works throughout the UK and the Republic of Ireland, although in only comparatively few centres. It was imported from the USA with the help of an organisation of the same name which has existed there for some years. Stop It Now! works to set up locally managed projects to raise awareness about child sexual offending. It produces and disseminates information and offers a helpline aimed at men and women who are worried about their sexual thoughts, feelings and behaviours regarding children; people who are concerned about the behaviour of someone close to them; and parents and carers and other adults worried about the behaviour of a child or young person.

In 2003–4 Stop It Now! had a target of 90 calls a month. It received 117 a month. The target was raised to 120 in 2004–5 and when this was achieved was raised to 150 calls a month in 2005–6. Eighty per cent of the calls come from the groups which Stop It Now! seeks to reach – abusers, potential abusers and their families – with 45 per cent of those coming from people who have committed an offence, or are worried that they may do so, or are distressed by their thoughts. (Stop It Now! does not say who the remaining 20 per cent of calls come from.) By May 2005, 4,000 calls had been taken and more than 2,000 individual callers had been helped. In addition, 250 people had been counselled by e-mail (Eldridge, Fuller, Findlater and Palmer no date).

Perhaps the most positive thing to emerge from Stop It Now! is the confirmation that there are people who are concerned about their thoughts, feelings and behaviour toward children and want to stop them. We know that treatment is available to only a few and we know that treatment, effective as it can be, is not a cure. However, Stop It Now! offers a preventative child protection service and recognises that child sexual abuse is not only a matter for the criminal justice, but is also a public health problem and that the responsibility for preventing it rests with the adults concerned.

As Stuart and Baines (2004) state: "The scale of the problem of sexual abuse of children is such that a major rethink of policy is needed – with much greater emphasis on prevention and early intervention." Much that has happened in the last 20 or so years – greater public awareness, advances in treatment and its greater availability – is welcome. However, the comparatively limited work of the kind offered by circles and Stop It Now!, the lack of residential facilities for treatment and, most of all, the extent of the sexual abuse of children, show that such recommendations remain aspirations.

The Men's Stories

Graham Byers

"You can work through it"

Graham Byers is 46 and for the past six and a half years he has lived with Cheryl Eliot, with whom he has a 3-year-old son, Gus. Graham has a 17-year-old daughter, Kim, from a previous relationship, although he has no contact with her. When he was in his 30s he abused his 7-year-old niece, an offence which Cheryl did not find out about until two years ago. He had received a two-year probation order. Two other offences were laid on file. In 2007 it emerged that, at about the same time as his first offence, he had abused another girl of the same age. He pleaded guilty to this and received a conditional discharge for two years, although, again, Cheryl did not know of this until the police came to their house. Graham says he lost his job as a result of the offence becoming public. At his own request, he has been on a sex offender programme, which lasts 180 hours. At the time of the interview he was a member of a relapse prevention group. He shows some talent as an artist and wants to set himself up as a self-employed decorator of custom cars, for which he has received a government grant. His first small exhibition was about to be mounted near where he lives.

Graham has attended two courses for his offending. He is an articulate man who appears to be deeply affected by the offences. He is also conscious of the damage which his deception has done to his relationship with Cheryl, with whom he says he wishes to speak more openly but for some reason finds it difficult to do so. He and his partner seem to have a different view about the state of their relationship: he believes that they are more successful in healing their relationship – he refers to it as "a success story" – than she will admit. Cheryl tells her story on page 93.

I'm from a large family, there's meself and I have three sisters, two brothers, and an extended family of cousins and aunties. Me mother, she's had a tough time and upbringing. She's the oldest of her three sisters and there's an age gap of about 10 years with her and the next one. Me grandma married again to a younger man about the same age as my mother, maybes a couple of years between them, which is what I was told later on in life. Me mother's husband, who was father to all the other children, used to frequently leave my mother and would come back later on. They would get back together and he'd then leave again and when me grandma's second husband came on the scene.

Obviously something had gone on between me mother and him, so up until the day he died I never knew. I thought he was me granddad, but he was me father: I was told this after the funeral by me grandma and me aunty.

Then I remember other things like when me brother got married we all went out and the man I thought was me father says, "Oh, it's great to be here with me two sons," and I was sat there thinking, "What about me then?" but I never put two and two together; I just thought, oh he's had a drink. I was sat on the other side with somebody and he put his arms around them and I always remember that, it always stuck in me mind and then obviously two and two went together.

From a very early age I was always going round to me grandparents' house, I always had a good bond with me granddad, more than any other one so I was round every single day. During the week I was round and then I ended up living there when I left school, going to college part time and doing me first job. I moved in 'cos he was very ill, he used to be on a nebulizer all the time and me gran couldn't look after him. I helped out till the day he died and then when I was told after the funeral, I says, "I was glad that he was."

Me father – I'll call me mother's husband that – was still alive and at me other brother's wedding, he came up to me and said, "I'm sorry to hear about your father," and I didn't want to make a scene or anything but I said why didn't you tell me? Like me mother to this day, she probably knows I know but I've never questioned her about it, so I never would raise it.

So it was weird but it wasn't weird in a way because I'd spent a lot of time with him, I had spent more time with him than anybody else so I felt I got … though I never got to call him dad, I called him granddad, but we had that bond as if we were son and father. Everyone knew except me but they didn't tell me until now, so, but I was pleased I had that bond with him that I did have, otherwise I think I might have gone demented.

This guy who I thought was me dad, I never saw much of him anyway 'cos when I was young (about 4 year old), me mam remarried, anyway, and he is me stepdad now but I just call him me dad 'cos he like brought us up anyway, like who I thought was me real father he was. He lived out of town anyway, he was out of the picture, but even though in here [taps his head] I thought he was me dad and if we ever went with me brother to go, he say, "I'm going to see me dad." But, yeah, me upbringing was just normal, just being a normal lad that I was.

I was born 1961 and [my first offence] was about 1994 or something like that. She was about 7 or 8. The period [when I offended] ran from about, say, 1991 to '95. There is six altogether of indecent assault, that's including this one that's just came forward. Four are on file and now I'm in my second year of a suspended sentence.

[*When did you come to some understanding about what your sexual interests were?*] Understanding – I think that would be the wrong word to use, 'cos I didn't understand otherwise I wouldn't have done it. If I'd understood it, used knowledge, wisdom, discernment I wouldn't have committed these offences.

I think my total thing was I was just satisfying lust, nothing more. I used to masturbate a lot and became dead after a while. I was looking for how can I satisfy my sexual lust and I didn't wake up one day and think "Ah, children." It was like I told the SBU [Sexual Abuse Unit], it was when I was round my brother's house I saw my niece – she was about 7 or 8 – she was just in a pair of knickers and I found myself turned on and I masturbated to it and then after that 'cos I enjoyed it. I didn't have any bad feelings or nothing and I used to go round a lot so like, as you do, you try to satisfy your sexual lust.

Obviously, there is something deranged about the way that you think, that's why when you say "understanding", I didn't understand it. Obviously, I wasn't like thinking as an adult, the way my actions were. There was something that had totally gone very, very wrong in my thinking to actually think it's okay to touch a child. It obviously wasn't.

When we do the risk factors [on the course], we do the relapse prevention, you have a risk swamp[1] and you put your name where you think you are on that risk swamp and I put myself as a low risk obviously. I mean, I could have said, "I'm wrong, I am never going to do it again, don't want to do it again," but up until the time that I did it, I didn't know I was going to interfere with children, young girls, so how can I say in the future – though I don't want to do it again – how can I say that? Though the likelihood, like I said, of me doing it again is minimal or none at all, none at all because of now what I know/understand, whereas before I didn't, I just went with my thoughts and bam! got caught, I got caught up in the cycle, but now I understand. I have a lot more knowledge/wisdom. I can use discernment in my decisions properly in life, but I do have to deal with it.

[*Having been through the course, what you have understood? How do you analyse your state of mind then and what do you think was happening to you?*] Oh yeah, I mean you have to look into the very embryo of yourself, you look into the murky depths of your mind 'cos I've listened to meself talking about it and it's strange but, like, I'll tape meself and through an MP3 player, ask questions and, like, role-play with meself and rewind and listen back. I just broke down, I just couldn't hack it what I was hearing ... what I was hearing 'cos all the time you're talking, you're just talking away to somebody but to actually just sit and listen and you're thinking to yourself, "Oh, my God."

I explained to the group what I had done, 'cos all the time you never get to hear what you're saying, you're talking, you're not like a listener, so I wanted to be a third party and listen to what I was saying at home, like role play and it was very weird actually listening to yourself and thinking, "Oh, my God, that's me."

What do I understand was going through me mind? As I say, I was just looking for something to satisfy me lust, it just so happened I chose children because when I was masturbating before ... in the end I was getting nothing, even thinking about me first wife, magazines – I was getting nothing and then I saw her in her knickers, very ... nothing to the imagination there. I found when I masturbated again I started thinking about that and it excited me more, so I thought, oh well, you do feel like you're doing nothing wrong, that's the state of mind you do actually get into, you do actually feel and believe that you are doing nothing wrong, you're not hurting anyone by doing this.

There was just like … I indecently assaulted … I used to read her bedtime stories and indecently assaulted this one, there was two where I hadn't indecently assaulted them, but I kissed them inappropriately, that was the other two and I indecently assaulted another one.

Yeah, it was always in the family, I mean I described myself as a wolf in sheep's clothing. It's the fact that I could walk about in the family, everyone knew me, they didn't know what was underneath waiting. Does that make sense?

At the time of the court case, the very first time it was the … you knew fine well … I had been caught and you know you don't ever want to do it … go through this and you do know it's about the children and it got … where it ended was that … they said because I was … I suffered a lot with anxiety back then, you just, you don't think about anyone else, you just think about yourself and you … everything's going through your mind and what have you done. I had forensic psychologists and all that talking to me. The next day I saw them again and I didn't even recognise him, he knew that, so what they said was they had come up with a deal to pleading guilty to this one, then the rest would go on file and they get suspended, and they says they're not doing it for you, we're doing it for the children and I says, "I understand," and that was the first time that I ever … that's what made me think about the children was when he said, "We're not doing it for you, we are doing it for the children," like bringing them back to court. So that made me think then. The first time I'd ever thought about what it did to the children was then and obviously during my probation we did an SBU but it wasn't in depth as this one, it just touched really lightly.

I thought I'd got off lightly, which I did. I got a three probation order. They [the course] go really in depth and they really make you look into yourself. The way I see it is that no matter what you do to a child, the courts decide the level of punishment to what you've done because they have guidelines in which to follow, but to the young child it's there no matter what punishment I get. What I've done to the child is the worst ever for them, even though you just say, "Oh, I've just touched them."

It's not something I've ever wanted to do before, it's simply that you wish that … obviously you don't want it to happen; you don't want it to happen again and you do want to push it to the back of your mind and not even think about it but when you're [on the course]. We [he and his partner] had to fight to get on this SBU, so what would be the point of going on it if I didn't … you know, there's no point saying all the right things that they want to hear without going really deep into your own mind otherwise you will get nothing out of it, you know.

[*When you were offending, did you ever talk to anyone, like a friend or GP?*] No because what it was – I don't know if you're familiar with the work that they do [on the course] – the cycle of offending where you do, like, intense feelings and what have you, justification and bad feelings, you know, in the cycle, I never ever did. I said I don't have any bad feelings, they says, "Well, why?" Then I explained that the very last offence that I committed was against Katie, my niece, I indecently assaulted her. She was asleep, or I thought she was asleep and I touched her and then she said "stop" and that is ... her voice was trembling, it was very difficult to hear the emotion in that voice and that was the only time I'd ever had bad feelings, 'cos they'd never have said nothing, 'cos in reality you want two things from that child – you want your sexual gratification from them and you want the silence, so you're not just asking for getting one thing, you want two things, even though I never threatened them or anything, you're just hoping that they don't say nothing and they didn't. It was only because of Katie, she's the last time I ever done touched, she I mean she said "stop" and I could really hear it in her voice, she said ... [At this point Graham stopped, very obviously overcome by the memory of what he was describing. After a minute or so he continued]. I still hear it now, it was really ... and if she hadn't said anything I'd have kept going, I know I would have 'cos what I did I enjoyed it, I can't lie about it.

You just hoped they wouldn't say anything but you want the silence, don't you? You know, you don't want to get caught, do you? You don't want to go through the court thing and everything, you don't want to be found out. I suppose with other crimes you don't want to be found out but with this, it's something you really, really don't want to get found out.

Katie moved. They live in Scotland now, they work up there, not because of me, it's just the way that things worked out. Her boyfriend and that got a job in Scotland. But like I say on that cycle, the bad feeling that might have kicked in because of what she said, but it's easy to see how the cycle works, how you do what you do and that's why I always think if you have a bad feeling about something, that affects you emotionally, how can you carry on? That's why I said I have never had any bad feelings about any of them, I just missed bad feelings and went straight to me next time like, looking forward to it, anticipation.

I wouldn't say all [justification] was absent because I would say to myself it was okay to do it. I wouldn't say it was completely missing but I didn't have to justify my bad feelings, because I didn't have any. I was justifying my actions, otherwise, like again, I wouldn't have done it if I didn't justify it, but justifying my bad feelings, I didn't have to because I didn't have any.

[*But you had married by this time, had relationships with women: how did they tie in with these feelings?*] It's something where you just throw [the impulse] away, you just don't even think about it. I didn't do it all the time, it was just like once and then eight months later again. The feelings and images that you get, you cannot just throw them away, they're always there, but it's how you control them rightly, you think about these images healthily or unhealthily but I always have Katie to remind me, when I talk about things. It ... just destroys me, I have to think what I've actually been a part of, but as regarding, like, in my relationships with adults and what have you, at that time I just swept it away, I didn't even think about it.

Ever since, if she [Katie] hadn't said "stop" and I felt bad it was as if a veil had been lifted or cataracts been removed and you could see everything clearly and you do question a lot about yourself. The first thing is, "Oh my God, what am I doing?" You do start to question yourself and ever since then I'd said that I would never do it again, I know I didn't want to again. Then, obviously, the court case and the SBU with the probation, we talked about it. Actually talking about it, I made sure, like certified, that I would never ever do it again and after that you just hope that everything goes the way you want it, just live a normal life. Then you find that it's very difficult 'cos before Cheryl, I'd had two relationships. They all just left their boyfriends for me even when they found out about everything. They said that they couldn't believe this. It wasn't, "I think you're dirty," or whatever. It was they couldn't, can't believe that I'd actually done something like that and they stayed with me, they still stayed with me, like the friends and family who knew about it and who all talked to me and that. I was glad that they won't just think, "Oh, you're all right, it doesn't matter," but it does matter. Like Cheryl detests it, she hates it. She will never forgive me and I hope she never does.

They accepted me, but they said they didn't like what I did and I am glad that they didn't like what I did otherwise it would be weird when I had met them and lived with them. After a time we split up and then this first one went back to their old boyfriend, so I don't know if I was a rebound case or what, but never mind, they didn't dump me straight away saying well, "I'm having nowt to do with you." They stayed with me 'cos they liked me as a person.

It was like having that whiteboard there [he points to a whiteboard on the wall of the room] and there's a blue dot in the corner and you can't help but see that blue dot because it stands out pretty much on a white background, but they still liked me and after that I met somebody else and she liked me. But there's always somebody out there ready to say, "Do you know what he's done?" and what have you, and she [the second relationship] confronted me about it and I said, "Yeah."

I says look, "If I had come out straight away and told you, you'd run faster than Lynford Christie." She says, "How would you know unless you asked me?" I says, "Well, I'm not going to take that chance." Maybes I should have told her but I didn't, but she stayed with me when she found out. I lived with her for about a year and a half but then things started to get a bit strained between us. But it was a normal relationship break-up and her boyfriend was on the scene quite a bit towards the end so I figured she wanted to get back with him, so that was that.

But the relationships I've been in, they've been still with me even though they'd found out, so that'd given me confidence if I did meet someone I would have to tell them later on, but then with the case with Cheryl I knew I had to tell her, but I couldn't because of what was happening with her son at that time. I thought "Oh my God, how am I gonna bring this up?" but then I had to bring it up because the police found out and that I was with her and I had to go and tell her.

Her son had been abused. She never told me but I could tell by just the way she talked with people on the phone and what have you – pick it up straight away – and 'cos of the actual work I'd done, from being very acute to what's being said and how things have been said. But I never questioned her about it, because I thought if she wanted to tell me, she would tell me, but I knew I had to tell her but I didn't know how. I really liked Cheryl and I knew that from me past two relationships that they still stayed with me even though they knew, so I knew that I could be confident enough to tell, but by the time I was gonna it was too late.

No, I didn't tell her about this one [the second offence] until it was too late. I had put it to the back of me mind so to speak. I had been to court for them and I sort of, like, thought that's it, otherwise I would have brought that up and it would have been left on a file with the rest unsaid if I'd told them then, that's what me lawyer said. I'd just completely blanked [the second offence] out of me mind and forgotten all about it.

I actually saw [the young woman] where I work and I thought, "Oh, flippin' heck," and then you're hoping again that she doesn't say anything because you don't want to go through it all again, but it was Cheryl's sister that she told and she said, "What do you think I should do?" Then her mam had rang me ex's sister, 'cos they all knew each other and then obviously they said "yes" and so she went to the police and the police came to the door. I knew what it was as soon as they said, so I went to the police station after work a few days later and I pleaded guilty straight away. After everything we've done, it obviously put a strain on me and Cheryl again and she was ready to throw me out, get rid of me.

She actually asked her 18-year-old son and if he'd have said, "I don't want him in the house," then I would have been gone, but she'd had a talk to him, obviously he likes me 'cos I'm still there.

[*How important do you regard Cheryl's relationship with you in helping you to deal with problems?*] Very important, very important. We should talk more about it to each other I think, more than what we do now. We have talked about it but not in any great depth. I would like to be able to talk to her about anything, like if I say in the future I feel I'm getting these urges again, I would like to think I would be able to talk to her about it, her talk to me. I feel that I could talk to her, but there is always people about, you know, we don't seem to have any time to ourselves, to really have an in-depth discussion like me and you are now. There is always somebody about, the kids awake …

I've never told her [about Katie] but I feel I should. She probably does know, but I've never actually sat down and put my view like, sat down in front of Cheryl and like I've talked to you now. We have talked about a lot of things but it's making sure that the opportunity's right, where we know what I'm on about.

From what I can gather I think that she thinks why does someone do what I did? She can't understand why, I mean I can't understand why a normal adult human being all of a sudden decides to just do that.

When I was on the course, Cheryl never used to ask all the time, if she didn't ask I wouldn't tell her basically because you used to come away quite drained from a session [on the Partners for Protection course] and it's not easy to do, it's difficult but well worth it. You come back drained and you come in and you tend to think, "Right, I've done that." You've thought about it all the way home and you feel like you just want a bit of normality back instead of having a full day there and driving back thinking, "Oh, I wish I said this now and I'll have to wait till next week," and you're chewing over it. You get home and see Gus and think it's nice homely atmosphere again and that's why I say I wish I could … I should have talked about it and say, "Right this is what we talked about." Some of the times we did 'cos like she knows some of the people there.

[*When I asked you why you agreed to meet, you said that it was to show it's not all doom and gloom and you talked about a success story. What do you mean by that?*] The first time the police and social services just said [to me and Cheryl], "Right, that's it, you have to split up," but why? Because there's kids involved, family and what have you. Like fair enough, so we didn't see each other, but Cheryl's solicitor said, "Why do you have to split up?" We want to prove to the officials that there can be a success story. It doesn't have to be because I've interfered with children, show that these courses do work you know, show that people like meself can get an understanding of what they've done wrong, why they've done wrong. It's not just like I say, "You know look at us, we're dead good 'cos we are doing this." It's not to show that. The way the social services are working, they would like it for me to leave and I feel it's because, "Oh, we don't have to worry about him any more, until he raises his ugly head again," but I want to show that you can work.

It's as a person, to prove to meself that, you know, if you want to do something, you can achieve this. You don't have listen to what they're saying in the papers or talk shows – these people are sick. Yeah, true but sick people can get better with the right help. Personally, for meself, it's not to stick two fingers up at the establishment, it's to show meself, show to Cheryl that something I did in that period of time obviously has great effect on everybody's lives and our lives as well, but you can work through it.

Now, I wouldn't put meself in some situations but when I go to the doctor's the quickest way, you have to go past a school. It doesn't bother me. It's like I be taking Gus to the nursery, we asked, they came round because I'm on the register again. I says, "Look, I'm taking Gus to school, he's going to nursery." No problem and so I think it depends on the institution again deeming how much of a threat they think you are.

What happened, happened in that time and there's been no others since then, you know. Well, of course, I couldn't go and be a volunteer, but that's the sort of thing where it wouldn't bother me anyways, I've never ever done it like that anyway, it's not something where I am going to suddenly start doing that. But, say, like for birthdays, he [Gus] wants some kids to come round, as I say I would like to be there but obviously if I can't be there, so be it. But it's like you say, the petty things will get ironed out in the future. I mean, if they thought I was such great a risk as that, how come I'm allowed to look after

Gus? So as far as that goes, I had a small success story in that part which the role's reversed: Cheryl goes to full-time work and I am hoping to work from home and be a dad to Gus, which is happening right now.

In the course, you have the same headings but it's what changed and you had to colour these like cheese wedges of how you have done. I'd split mine in half 'cos there was like "inner peace". I only coloured half way on all of them but other ones like "knowledge" and that and stuff I coloured in whole. But where you talk about like yourself and what have – your peace, how you are – that I could only colour say half in. I don't think I'll ever have inner peace with regard to what I've done. I'll never get over that. I don't think the young children will either. I haven't got complete inner peace, I don't think I ever will.

I'm never, ever judgemental. On the course, we were there to help each other. When I listened to them [other course participants], if I didn't feel any emotion by what they were doing and you thought, "Well I never did that," that's maybes the only time I am glad I wasn't like that, 'cos I feel bad enough now – how would I have felt then? This other guy, who had been in prison for 18 years, you can imagine what he might have done. He was still locked up when he was coming to the group, but I was glad that I wasn't like that but I didn't say. It's like we had someone who was a flasher but you weren't there to say, "Is that all you did? What you doing here?"

I was always forthcoming in what I said because I knew why I was there, some of them held back and you could tell so. Rather than the two group leaders there, it was our job to get it out of them and so while you were trying to get it out of them you were looking at yourself as well. Very clever the way it was done, so you didn't really have the time really to think of judging someone.

The first few weeks was difficult because you were talking to somebody about what you done but when you do your personal work you have to stand up and you have to go through it and then by what you have written there's a lot of other stuff gets added in. The best questions sort of end in me talking about indecently assaulting my niece. Well what did you do? Oh, right I did this, and then they will ask questions to make you think about your own actions. It was very difficult that first one and then with the next one we all knew what was coming so we'd be more open and honest, because at first you tend to hold back. We all did but then that wasn't the reason why we were there and then that's why you stand up and do your personal work even though it was difficult. Everyone fires questions and it makes you really think.

If there was something in the past, I think I would know. I think the only way is to reach into the depth, but up until that time when I offended, I had never done nothing – anything – like that before. I mean, everything has a beginning, doesn't it somewhere along the line? So whether it was 30 years ago or 30 years later, it had a beginning. It had to start somewhere. I dunno you can talk for ages, can't you about it all?

Paul Carpenter

"I'd like someone to confide in"

Paul Carpenter is 29. He is dressed in a tracksuit top and combat trousers. He is personable but has obvious difficulty in relating his story: he moves around, somewhat agitatedly, on his seat; sometimes he slumps back, sometimes he sits forward. His physical discomfiture betrays emotions. He often pauses in mid sentence and when he speaks at length he often hesitates. He describes his family as middle class – his mother is a senior teacher, his father an engineer – but quickly adds, "I'm not living a middle-class life." He works in a warehouse ("it's a bit more than the minimum wage") and lives in the Dales. He spent a year training as a nurse but dropped out, partly because of problems with a relationship and partly because he found the academic work difficult. Paul is unusual among offenders. Becoming increasingly acutely conscious that what he was doing was wrong, he went to the police and confessed to his offence. There was no trial as it was thought that the child's evidence would not hold up in court. Paul regrets that he has not been punished for his offences. He went to his GP and was referred to a psychiatrist. He was later assessed and went on a course for sex offenders.

Right, I've got one sister, she's three years younger. I born in 1978 in Leeds, and then since I was a baby, we lived in the same house in the Dales in a village, a small village, went to a little village school, then a sort of small-town comprehensive. Since I left school I've tried a few college courses and stuff and I've had quite a few jobs which I haven't stuck at for very long for various reasons and then, more recently, I've sort of started sticking at things a bit better. I suppose, you know, 'cos I wanted to get a more stable life, have a bit more money and stuff.

A lot of [me childhood] was good. I had some good friends and some good times. When I first went to see the doctor about me sexual behaviour problem, I was looking back on me childhood and trying to look for things, like if I had been abused in any way or anything sort of unusual that might have affected how I came to have this kind of dysfunction, but I can't really remember anything like that. But I sort of still kinda, somehow I believe that it kind of, like, it somehow started when I was a child; that's just me opinion probably.

I have memories of me mum being quite cruel to me [as a child]. I have to look at it objectively from me point of view now, but I feel that she was –

whether intentionally or not. Like, if you did something naughty, she wouldn't tell me, you know, "Don't do that," she would say, "You're a bad child and you embarrass me, you're an embarrassment in front of our friends," and stuff, which probably a lot of parents say, but I can remember taking it to heart and thinking, "All right, I am a bad person." Me dad was, from what I can remember, sort of quite timid and me mum used to be the kind of the … the woman scared me.

One of the biggest regrets of me life was I used to bully me sister. She was three years younger and I used to hit her and be mean to her and all sorts of stuff and that was from when I was really young. I believe it was because I was having some problem with possibly me mum that was causing me to have that anger. It was more than your normal brother–sister fighting. I used to, like, do proper punching and stuff. I used to keep on bullying her and she used to get her own back. She found a way of coping with it by not fighting back, but sometimes lying to me mum and dad that I had done bad stuff to her and I hadn't, as a way of fighting back, so I would sometimes get told off and I hadn't done anything.

Then, when I was about 15 she was about 12, I was watching TV and I flipped the channel over onto something I wanted to watch and she grabbed the remote control and threw it at me, threw it at me head really hard. I sort of grabbed her and threw her to the floor and I sort of stomped on the back of her head and her face, smashed a cereal bowl all over the floor and something just cracked in me and I just thought, "What the hell's going on here?" and we never had another fight again. Things are okay between us now, we talk and stuff but, you know, it must have been really bad for her at the time.

With me sexual behaviour, I can remember we had family friends who had two daughters: one was about my age and one was about six years younger. I remember we went on holiday with them. I think I was about 16 and she was 10 and I remember sort of doing something inappropriate, kind of, like, what I know now is grooming behaviour and possibly before that as well, like playing games where I would be becoming aroused by the physical contact but she wasn't aware of it.

We used to get on quite well, she liked me so I used to like think that, you know, I am playing with one of me friends but really I would be sort of trying to get into a situation where I would be, like, touching her in the game and kind of just, you know, playing around wrestling or something, but not so she would know that it was a sexual thing to me.

Before that – this would be when I was about 11 or 12 – I remember where instead of wanting to talk to girls and then get to know them and hold their hands and stuff, I would be wanting to touch them in a situation without them sort of being aware I was doing it.

I have always been attracted to girls me own age and now sort of women me own age, as well as having this problem. At the time, I wasn't aware what it was, that I had a problem at all, not until I was in me 20s. I think I just mentally blocked it and I never thought that this is a problem, although I think it did feel like a problem, but for some reason I didn't think about it at all.

It changed from being sort of an unconscious thing that I was doing and I blocked to me starting to do it more and think about it more, kind of like looking at girls that were young and thinking sexual thoughts. And worse: grooming behaviour I was doing up until me 20s. It's sort of sophisticated grooming strategies but for young girls and trying to get situations where they trust me and like me and then I sort of touch them sexually but without them realising that I was doing it and making it into a game.

I realised there was something wrong quite a way before I went to the doctor. I think I was about 23 and it was shortly after the worst sort of grooming sexual assault I'd done. I was renting a room off a woman in Ripon and her granddaughter used to come and stay. She was 10 or 11 and she'd come and talk to me so I engineered the situation where I'd be playing games with her and stuff. For example, like telling her it would be a game for her to try and not let me lift her off the floor, which obviously is impossible. Then I'd try and lift her off the floor so I could touch her between her legs and keep it a game so she wouldn't say anything.

I was fully aware that it was wrong and it was then that I was more seriously doing it, doing the worst kind of things. Then after that, one night I got really drunk and I told one of me friends about it but he was drunk as well and he didn't tell me until I went to the doctor that I told him. I didn't realise but he said it was too much for him to deal with; he just kind of ignored it. I can understand that.

I went to the GP and he referred me to a psychiatric doctor in the hospital and I went to see this psychiatrist and he talked it through with me on a couple of occasions and said, after the end of it, sort of, "In terms of mental health, this isn't like a mental health illness you've got but, obviously, it is a problem." He was saying, "What do you think your options are?", and I said, "Well, I suppose, I can go to the police or just try to carry on with trying not to do it or look for alternative treatments or something." He said, "Yeah, that's probably your best bet." He said that's all he could do and I was quite devastated 'cos I'd managed to go to see him. It had helped to talk to a real doctor but not much had happened.

I thought, "This is serious," and as I didn't get a serious enough reaction or response, I decided to go to the police and just describe the worst sort of case of sexual abuse I'd done. So I went to local police station and told them. I said, "I'm a paedophile," and listed what I'd done and they arrested me. Me parents had no idea at this point so the first they knew was the police turned up at the house and took away a computer so that was an awful moment for them. They came down to the police station and after being interviewed by a detective I got bailed. They interviewed the little girl whose testimony … well, her memory of it was insufficient for a charge so it never went any further than that.

I actually feel it would have been better for me – it's maybe a kind of martyrish thing to think – to have some form of punishment. It doesn't sit right with me that, I'm just sat in a room with some really nice people like [staff on the sex offenders' course] and they've been helpful but I've done something wrong, something really wrong and there's been no kind of punishment. I don't mean probably being with lots of people in a normal prison 'cos that could possibly cause more harm than good to me, like too much for me to deal with, but perhaps being locked up somewhere. I know that would be more expensive for the taxpayer. Just kind of while all this process was taking place, it might have been better to put me in some sort of secure unit. Me close friends think of me as someone who reproaches meself. I suppose I get a lot of negative thoughts about meself and anxiety and sort of depression and seeking to be alone because I don't want to make other people's lives worse by me being there, which isn't helpful behaviour. There's a part of me that just feels like bad about meself.

It felt it was like the right thing to do [going to the GP and the police], yeah, and it seems really helpful. You know, I wish I had talked to someone a lot earlier but at that point, when I did manage to go to me doctor, that was the right thing to do and it was a lot better to do it then than wait until I got caught or something.

Most of the focus of the [sexual offenders'] course [I attended] was on practical ways to avoid hurting children, like real behavioural techniques and exercises to stop me thinking about that kind of thing; that's what most of it was. It wasn't really something that they got to the root of – of why I was like that, so that's still kind of on me mind sometimes.

I think the main help [with the course] is getting past the twist in me head that was thinking of the justifications, that it wasn't actually hurting anyone and stuff. That was just sort of seeing it for what it was, this kind of grooming and leading on to hurt, violation: do you believe the child's consenting because they're not objecting? They're not ready for those kinds of thoughts or feelings.

I felt too bad to talk to anyone really, although, as I said, I had mentioned to me friend when I was younger. Me mum and dad? A little bit, but it wasn't very good because me mum tried to convince me that I hadn't really done anything; it was just she couldn't cope with it. She was saying, "You haven't really done anything." She wanted to think that I had kind of made it up because she thinks I'm sort of, like, a bit of a martyr type, which I do feel sometimes a little bit, but in this case it was unhelpful 'cos I actually needed people to sort of take me seriously and not say it's not as serious as you think. I don't remember [my father] really saying anything. He seems, maybe, per-plexed, I don't know. Thinking about it, it's kind of weird but I don't think he really said anything.

Me mum was saying, "You make it more serious than it is, you haven't really done anything wrong," and me dad, I remember him not saying any-thing unhelpful, like he didn't say anything melodramatic like, you know, "You're not me son," or anything. He didn't take it as serious.

I suppose I never thought of it that way [that it was strange that my parents have still not discussed with me what happened]. Me mum seemed to never really take it in properly. I don't know how she has it in her head now. I think me dad sort of comprehended it a little better. He's never talked to me about it since, and I'm not sure, I'm not sure why. I mean, I presume it's 'cos they find it hard to broach the subject and I haven't really wanted to talk to them about it.

I rang [my sister] to tell her and it freaked her out. Oh, yeah, I forgot to say this earlier but just before I went to the doctor, me sister had been away on a gap year and she come back and she'd had some kind of illness and me mum and dad didn't know what it was. They took her to the hospital. She was having like coughing fits and she would go really quiet and wouldn't say anything for hours. Then one night she told me that when she had been in Thailand and she had been attacked by two men, been dragged down the street and they had raped her. This was a couple of years after it happened but me mum and dad still don't know, which I find really hard. It shocked me. It was quite soon after that, that I went to the doctor. I think hearing about a sexual assault on a woman that I cared about, helped me to see what I was doing from the point of view of the parents of the little girl, the victim, so it's a really awful thing to hear about but, it kind of like ... it had in a way a positive effect on me.

Yeah, I went to a relapse prevention group. I went back to the GP (a different one), and she referred me to the group and I went for an interview so they could establish what treatment ... if any I needed. I went straight into the end of the last group rather than doing the whole thing because it was felt I had already got past that stage where you are in denial about it.

Before I went to see [professionals] I knew I had a really serious problem which could end up with me seriously hurting a child or me going to jail or just bad outcomes, but I hadn't realised that what I was doing was grooming. I had a twist in me head and I thought it was just kind of happening, I didn't realise it was me doing it all, I just thought it was just happening and I couldn't stop it.

At the time it was a lot like that with me [justifying what I was doing by saying that the child would like it or didn't mind]. It was actually, "The girl wants me to touch her like this and she enjoys it." I thought thoughts like this could develop further into a sexual relationship but it wouldn't actually be harmful and it wouldn't be rape or anything, it would be like boyfriend and girlfriend and I would be, like, 22 and this would be a 10- or 11-year-old girl or younger. Me grooming never got past that stage but I had a lot of sexual fantasies about taking it further but some part of me held back. I think that was the part of me that was worried about getting caught rather than any good part of me.

I'm not sure [if I was stopped for fear of hurting a child] 'cos I believe that the grooming and the sexual touching is hard for any [child], so I was kind of hurting. I am not the kind of person that would do something that would cause a child physical pain, but what I was doing was, well, sort of violating them in a way. Dealing with the consequences, I could delude meself that everything was fine, but I wouldn't be able to cope with, like, actually forcing them to do anything but I wouldn't ... I don't think I ... I don't know ... I never did that anyway.

Since I went to the police I've told me mum and dad and sister and I've probably talked to the friend I talked to before (when I was drunk). He wasn't particularly helpful this time either, but he's a really good friend and we are still good friends. Really, it's just he didn't say anything; he didn't really have much reaction at all.

Me other friend that I told, he had what I would call the most normal reaction – he was just really shocked and said he was disgusted and he thought I was disgusting. He walked out and then at some point after that he talked to me and said, "I think it's a good thing you went to the police," and we are good friends again now. That whole reaction I considered to be the most sort of normal, or not normal but, you know, just a good reaction from a good person.

Then also the guy [Herb] who was living in the house with me when I was doing the abuse in Ripon. A while later I also told me friend I was then sharing a house with 'cos since I was sharing a house with him it would be better to tell him.

The friend [Herb] I am living with now, he just found it a bit hard to take in and didn't really say much. I haven't really talked about it much since, so I'm not sure. I'm not close friends with him. It's just with us sharing a house so I thought I better tell him.

There's a part of me feels more comfortable being around people who are aware of the worst thing I've done, rather than people having a higher opinion of me than what I actually am. That's another thing me mum said to me. She was really, really against me telling me sister and talking to me friends about it. I explained to her that I needed to tell a couple of people close to me and she was really trying to persuade me not to tell anyone, which I can understand from her point of view, but it wasn't helpful to me.

With me mum there's a lot of stuff I am not sure about. I do know that she was adopted and she doesn't know who her real parents are and I believe that she had some problems. I know she had post-natal depression when I was born and I believe she maybe had some unresolved psychological issues when I was a very young baby, but I obviously don't know that for sure. I think possibly there's been some moments when I was young when she's either taken out problems in her life on me just in anger or something, or there's stuff that I don't even know about but that's more just a hunch. In fact, I do have these memories of her really badly losing her temper and telling me stuff about "You're a bad person," but I think it's hard for me to be objective about it.

When I was a teenager me confidence went really down. There was a girl at school when I was about 17 and she was 17 and we sort of got together at a party and started kissing and stuff and then it never worked out but I had a massive obsession with her for about a year or two. At the time I was smoking a lot of marijuana and drinking a lot and experimenting with a lot of other drugs as well and … and for this reason, I got quite depressed. I think, looking back on it, people around me thought it was just a teenage phase, which it partly was.

Me first sexual experience, the first time I had sex, was with an older woman. She was 37 and I was 19. It just didn't feel right. She was married, she was our next-door neighbour. I used to go round to the house sometimes. Me and me sister would go round because they [the woman and her husband] were a bit younger than me mum and dad. They used to say to go round and have a beer with them. But then she probably flirted and she gave me a secret letter saying she liked me. I've ... I've found out since that she has had another affair with a man closer to her own age. I think for her it was just kind of boredom and an unhappy marriage but for me it was ... it just wasn't right. It wasn't terrible, it just didn't feel right. I kind of, like, had to almost force meself to do it because I thought, "Right, I need to start having sex with women," and I think she was worried that I wouldn't find her attractive and I just felt ... I don't know. We ended up having sex a few times but I didn't enjoy it basically. It kind of, like, maybe in a small way might have put me off having sex with women or something. I don't know, but it's not a large factor in the thing though. Now, I get drunk and have one-night stands after night clubs.

There was one other time with a married woman who was me own age, who I really, really liked a lot but she didn't leave her husband. We were on a nursing course together. We actually never really had sex ... well, we kind of had sex a couple of times but it was mainly sort of making out 'cos she felt guilty 'cos she didn't want to do it, but, you know, it seems she actually didn't want to cheat on he husband but she liked me. Yeah, I really, really liked her; it went on for months. She was a student nurse like me. She was from a Bangladeshi family and she told me she was married pretty early on but I didn't believe her because she hadn't changed her surname. I think she might have had a marriage that was legal in Bangladesh but not legal in England; it's really complicated.

Yeah, yeah, it must be [that my ability to form relationships with women is complicated by my sexual attraction to children]. Yeah, in a kind of obvious way and in more subtle ways I think, like, if people pick up on things. I can probably seem sometimes uncomfortable with meself and the women would pick up on that and think, "Why?" They won't know what it is but they'll think there's something not right there and it's a large factor, an obstacle in trying to form relationships with women.

One of the big [obstacles to having a relationship] is that I feel like I'm not worthy of sort of being loved, so that doesn't help to start with. Then I've also got (I don't know if that's it) low sexual confidence and I think that the woman will, you know ... If I had sex with a woman I think "this is not much for a man" kind of thing. I always felt that it's unhelpful, that it's actually feeding into this problem I have. I need to overcome these negative thoughts if I'm gonna have a happy, offence-free life.

I don't think there is actually any real problem there with me having a relationship with a women apart from it's kind of, like, phantoms in me head kind of thing. It is there on the horizon. If I want to have a serious relationship with someone there is the sort of worry of them finding out about this problem or me having to tell them if they want to have children. I mean, I am not sure whether I would have to tell them, but I think I would want to if it is going to be a worthwhile relationship. I think if I didn't it would be a bit of like two people who had sex without actually knowing each other.

I have got friends who have got children and stuff like that can cause problems. If it is friends like Herb, me friend who lived in the house with me in Ripon when the abuse happened, his girlfriend has a young son and he's 5, so I've kind've got to know him through being friends with Herb and his girlfriend. But it's okay now because he [Herb] knows about me past, he won't let me get into a situation where I was on me own with the boy and it's never a problem, it's fine. I don't know how much his girlfriend knows – that's for him to decide – but that feels awkward to me because I'd pretty much rather she knew.

I used to look for situations like where I would be closer to young girls and now I try not to. I'm not fully there on it, on that side of it, I'm still, like, kind of like the … you know, the roots are still there, whatever it is, which means that I could still find meself headed back towards those kind of behaviours, but the difference being now, I'm not in denial about it.

I suppose I'm actually going back in me head; it's more in the mindset or something, I mean the inappropriate sexual fantasies. I haven't really mentioned that, that's actually a big part of the treatment as well, like stopping the masturbating to only think about consenting women, not about, you know, schoolgirls and stuff. I have got to agree that's really important and that's the hardest thing because it's only fantasies in the head. That's the hardest thing to control.

I was managing to just either think about women in me life or using magazines (you know, a *Playboy* or something like that) and it's going really well but I've had like a … I got a bit difficult with it recently. It's hard to talk to [a female staff member] about it actually 'cos I find it a lot easier to talk to [a male psychiatrist who had worked with him] about it, but I'm not on his programme any more so I can't talk to him, well I suppose I could ring him, I just, I just … I'll possibly write to him or something. The thing is, it's things I've already said to him before, it's nothing new, it's just that at the time when I've seen him I've managed to totally eradicate it, but since I've finished the programme it's sort of creeping back. When I was … when I was taking me class [the course] I was taking anti-depressants as well and they were helping and I chose to come off them and since I have come off them I think it has become more difficult to sort of stop meself slipping back into it.

Talking to you actually helps a lot. It's good to be able to say it to you actually, you know, because I don't have anyone to talk to. I mean I've got friends I've told but I don't feel like I can talk to them on a weekly basis about how I'm feeling. I can make stupid errors because I've got no way of seeing the obvious things I need to do.

Even when I've been kind of in love with a woman me own age and she likes me – actually, I'm talking about before I went on the [sex offenders'] programme – I would still be having inappropriate sexual thoughts as well and

I saw young girls. I'm not so sure now 'cos I've got more practical skills and knowledge to help me avoid it but, yeah, that is a problem not having someone. I can talk a little bit about the little problems and it sometimes means that I end up not dealing with them and also means it could end up with me committing another offence if I let it come to me like that.

I managed totally to cut out having fantasies, sexual fantasies about children, and then, gradually, it started again. I was really drunk one time and I decided to masturbate but, for whatever reason, I slipped into the old pattern of thinking about a schoolgirl rather than a woman, then I didn't have anyone to … I could have rung [the psychiatrist] or talked to me doctor about it but I didn't. I think I actually did tell [the female Mosaic staff member] and eventually I brought it up in the group. They said, "It's good that you brought it up," and I think I said I was gonna agree to be able to come to the next group and say how everything was. It wasn't for a couple of months again and I managed to avoid the inappropriate fantasies, but that's the problem: it seems I let it get back in there and that's the hardest thing.

Yeah, I've thought about it [his drinking having an effect on fantasising]. I still drink quite a bit so I probably get pissed one night on the weekend. I think it probably would help if I cut down on it, and that's one of the things that I did talk to [the psychiatrist] about a bit and I think, for me, he thought that drinking was not a major issue.

I've never really excelled in any job I've done. I've had some with some things that I'm good at. There's been jobs in shops and factories and warehouses and things like that. I did a bar job for a bit. With the nursing course, I was struggling with the written side of it. I'm poor at writing. I can count with me hands but I can't type and I sometimes find it hard to be clear when I talk as well. I'm fine reading and listening to people, but for some reason I find getting words out in any form doesn't come naturally to me. I can understand what you're saying but I am not that clear when I try and talk. So, it was partly that and partly 'cos when I was there I had a really bad time with Aisha [the married fellow student].

It's one of me regrets that I think without the problems I've had I would have really enjoyed something like teaching, which I can't do that now. Or I'd have liked to have done something like being a paramedic, but obviously I can't do that either.

In this job I'm doing at the moment, I get on okay with other people but it's not particularly good money – it's a bit more than minimum wage – and I can just about do the job. I'm not naturally good at writing, as I said, and also me concentration's not very good. I kind of daydream a lot, so although in certain ways I'm sort of fairly intelligent, I haven't managed to find a way of putting that into a career.

I went to a career counsellor and he came up with photography, which I'd thought about but I wouldn't want to do like, the small-time photographing weddings and things like that, partly 'cos I wouldn't want to be photographing children, and even with the parents there, it just wouldn't feel right. I dunno, I might be taking it a bit far by thinking like that but I just would rather not do a job that involves children at all.

I think I'd like having a girlfriend who I could sort of like confide in and stuff. It would be really good and I do have a shower every day and put on a decent T-shirt but I'm not into clothes and stuff like that, but not all girls, all women are.

Where I live, it's a small town and the women in their 20s who have stayed there, have only stayed there 'cos they've settled down, and the women who have moved away have gone to university or gone off on careers, so you find young women, 20–30, have mainly already married or got long-term relationships. So that's not ideal, but I haven't got particularly anywhere else to go. A couple of friends live there and it's near where me mum and dad live – they live in a village about seven miles away – and I just kind of ended up back there. I don't particularly like the place.

Ripon was fair but I probably wouldn't go back to Ripon 'cos I've got this association: the little girl's family still live there and it mightn't be … I might get paranoid, or not even paranoid, it just might not be safe for me, but I think I would be better off socialising in a bigger place, where I do meet women, but especially not somewhere I went to school.

4   A place of safety

Jesmond is an attractive and self-contained area only three stops on the Metro from Newcastle's central railway station. It is a place of handsome, mainly red-brick, mid-Victorian and Edwardian terraced houses, where even a modest two-bedroom flat can fetch £270,000 and a substantial, three-storey family home £750,000. A collection of small streets, lined with mainly local shops, not far from one of the area's two Metro stations, gives it the distinct feel of a self-sufficient urban village. To walk its long main street, which runs roughly between the two stations, is to run a gauntlet of small hotels, bars, cafes and restaurants. This is an area populated by professionals but where numerous "To Let" signs also betray its popularity with students. All that prevents it being the Left Bank of Newcastle is the lack of a cinema: the white-brick former Jesmond Cinema is now in sad decay, with weeds sprouting from its upper reaches.

Situated unobtrusively amid this very typical example of late twentieth-century/early twenty-first-century revitalised, fashionable urban living is the headquarters of Barnardo's Mosaic project, a tall house, once a spacious family home. It sits slightly set back from the road, with only a plaque by the door to distinguish it from its neighbours. This modesty belies its work. In fact, it is one of probably only three projects in the UK working specifically with women whose families have been affected by abuse and maybe the only one catering for the female partners of child sex offenders. Formed in 1994 as the Family Resource Service (it took its present name in 1996), Mosaic also works with women in other situations. The Family Resource Service was initially a specialist part of Barnardo's fostering and adoption service, which found placements for children who had been abused. It began working with the probation service and the Sexual Offenders Treatment Group, working with offenders to develop empathy with their victims. Its present work came about through the realisation that there was no therapeutic service for partners of the men in the groups. The assumption had been that that was the role of the social services departments. At this time the Sexual Behaviour Unit – created by the Newcastle, North Tyneside and Northumberland Mental Health NHS Trust and the National Probation Service Northumbria – was starting to work with men who had abused children but who were not in the criminal justice system.

It was this realisation that led Mosaic and the Sexual Behaviour Unit to create a joint initiative in 1995, the Partners for Protection programme, intended to assess the capacity of the mothers who attended to protect their children from abuse. The programme aims to identify "a woman's capacity to move from their position in an 'offender-organised' system to a more protective position in a 'child-centred' system" (Clothier 2008: 12). Ninety women have attended the programme to date (September 2008).[1]

Smith (1994) has identified ten areas which are thought to contribute to a non-abusing parent's capacity to protect. They are:

- how a mother responds to her child's disclosure of abuse
- a mother's feelings toward her child following disclosure
- the part a mother had in the disclosure process
- who she feels is responsible for the abuse
- her perceived options
- the extent to which she cooperates with statutory agencies
- the history of her relationship with her partner
- how willing she is to discuss sexual abuse
- her own history of abuse (if any); and
- how vulnerable she may be by virtue of other matters like, for example, disability.

The programme attempts to be sensitive and non-judgemental and a place where women are listened to. This, in itself, will be novel for some of those who attend. It aims to:

- provide education and increase awareness of the many issues concerned with abuse;
- facilitate experiential development through emotional expression and improved self-awareness;
- create a supportive environment to foster self-empowerment; and
- facilitate the development of self- and child protection.

A Partners for Protection group is now run by a male and female co-worker so that it is always evident how people of each gender should behave toward each other. Each group is held for six hours, one day a week for eight weeks. Each group has a maximum of eight members and activities include work in small groups, video, individual work and discussion, with exercises, role play, role reversal and sculpting. (Sculpting is where family dynamics are pictured through either role play or the use of materials like toys or stones and shells.) Experiences are shared through the creation of life maps (a pictorial representation of the woman's life until the present). To help women to understand more fully about sexual abuse, sessions are devoted to the effects of child sexual abuse and how children can be talked to about sex. There are also sessions on managing disclosure; models of offending; family perspectives; and creating safe environments. While some sessions offer information, they are not detached from group members' own experience but are also intended to help them to see the relevance of what they are learning to their own experiences and how they can now move forward.

To attend, a woman must be aged 18 and over. Those with mild learning disabilities may be admitted but sometimes struggle with the concepts and methods used. Support is offered to any participants who have difficulty with reading and writing. Female abusers are excluded and women with acute mental health problems may be excluded if they are thought likely to be disruptive.

The one session I attended was the last of the course for its five members. When asked how each felt about its being the last meeting, all said they were pleased the course had come to an end but were uniformly positive about what it had meant to them:

> It's gone really well – I think I've done really well. It's all come together and gone the way I wanted it to go.
>
> I've enjoyed coming, I always looked forward to coming and I've learned a lot. It's a bit of a disappointment that it's finishing. I didn't want to come at first – I'm not someone who'd want to be in a group, but that's different now.
>
> I'm pleased it's over but I'll miss it. It's been something for me, not for the kids and [partner]. I always felt that I was making excuses for him, that I had to stick up for him but I don't feel that I have to do that now. Now I have the little 'uns who need me and [partner] is big and ugly enough to look after himself.
>
> I'm pleased it's come to an end. It's taken its toll on me, though I'll miss the lassies, obviously.

Brief though my experience of the group was, it was still obvious how the women had been able to come to a new understanding of their circumstances through an enhanced insight into their own lives and through the prism of the experiences of the others. This had very obviously effected a shift in their perspectives.

Few of the women who took part in this group had any real contact with their partners. This was true of those in other groups and of the women whom I interviewed. For a couple of women who did still have contact, it was extremely distant, reduced, in one case, to the occasional short telephone conversation.

The most up-to-date research into the Partners for Protection programme was conducted by Hill (2003). By August 2003, 14 women had completed the programme, 8 in the first group and 6 in the second. Their average age was 34.4 years (range 25–46 years). All were white Caucasian, which reflects the local population (although group members come from areas a good distance from Newcastle) and health service referrals. All had children who ranged in age from 1 to adolescence. At the start of the group, 10 women had children living at home, and 2 others had children returned to them from care during the course of the group. Only four of the women's children were known to have been abused, but in most cases the risk was posed by the woman's present or recent partner. (In one case the risk stemmed from the woman coming from a family of incestuous relationships.)

Five women in Hill's study were cohabitating at the time (four of them with known abusers) and three went on to develop relationships, some with men felt to pose a risk. One woman wanted to restart her relationship with her husband, a known abuser. Of the women who were separated, six had other problems: for two there was domestic violence; for another emotional abuse; and in four cases there was neglect of their children. Two of the women were assessed as having borderline learning disabilities and required help to complete some of the tasks in the programme. Another woman had cerebral palsy. Most of the women were receiving state benefits, although three were in paid employment. Two of those worked part time.

> No woman commented upon adverse financial impoverishment as a result of her relationship breakup, most feeling that they could manage well enough on state benefits, although obviously money could be tight with children to provide for also.
>
> (Hill 2003: 3–4)

The course is carefully crafted to make sure that the learning methods used are appropriate to those attending, that assessment is built in, and that the therapeutic environment in the group is conducive to change. The groups are also posited on the idea that group members gain more where there is a balance of "support" and "challenge" built into the group's operation. These come from the facilitators, who encourage that the women themselves should offer support and challenge to each other.

Something of the women's initial reactions is described by Hill (2003):

> Managing group processes was one of the most difficult tasks for group workers. Initially, a lot of time was needed to process the women's anger, mistrust, hurt and disbelief at what had happened to them, including their journey so far with professional agencies. There was a strong perception of injustice in needing to attend such a group when they hadn't done anything wrong. (p. 4)

Carrie (not her real name) probably speaks for many women when she says:

> I came strictly with my arm up back. I didn't want to come and I don't think that any woman did.
>
> (Mosaic 2002)

Hill reports that group workers found (as researchers have done) that the women expressed anger toward their children, attributing the abuse as "innocent" or even fabricated. But, she notes, "such emotions are not coherent, continued emotional states, rather only a proportion of a confused, rapidly changing kaleidoscope of emotions more akin to chaos" (Hill 2003: 4). Indeed, "There was no evidence in any of the women of disinterest [*sic*] toward their child's suffering, only of extreme confusion, initial disbelief and nowhere helpful to turn" (ibid.: 5).

The programme has also developed for women other than those with an offending partner so that, for example, it is available to those with a son or father who has abused.

Referrals come from courts and local authority children's services departments (and formerly from social services departments) when there may be doubts about women's protective ability: the likelihood that they will be vulnerable to being used by another potential partner to reach their child. In these cases, attendance can be a key factor as to whether a woman keeps her child or (if the child is in care) whether her child is returned to her. All but one of the women who have attended the Parents for Protection programme have completed the course, although it is not something that many women take to willingly when their attendance is stipulated by the courts or the local authority.

Carol Butler, Project Manager, Mosaic, points to the emotional importance of the programme for some of the women: "It's sad that an assessment can be a quality time when they've been listened to and that's never happened before" (Butler 2007).

Because of their role in child protection, staff working in the programme could come to be seen by mothers as "another agency", engendering consequent distrust. However, the opposite has proved to be the case: the work has been seen by some as giving them an authority and power which they have never previously known, an additional belief in themselves and a strength not hitherto enjoyed. One woman had her children returned from care largely as a result of the role she had played in the group and the voice which she had found there. When this voice was heard by other agencies, she gained a sense of power and control (Hill 2003: 5).

For some attendees there is an element of coercion about their attending initially, but the service is independent of all other agencies like police and social services. Again, Carrie: "We felt that we could trust all the staff and the other women. No one would be judgmental" (Mosaic 2002).

Ann Baker, a mother interviewed for this book, said:

> I did come and I was nervous on the first day but, honestly, it was the best thing I have ever done. It's just opened my eyes to what can happen. It's changed me, it's changed me a lot because I was always very soft with people, I couldn't see no bad in anybody and that's toughened me up, going on this course. I've learnt a lot and that's what I'm saying: I know now what my husband was doing to me, while he was abusing my daughter. It's been really good, it's a really good course to go on. With

others like me on the course, it was better for me because I honestly didn't think I would be able to speak out or join in anything because I am very shy and quiet and they couldn't believe it when I said I was quiet, because I wasn't. I shocked meself, but I got on with everybody. All the women were brilliant, really nice, and it was nice for me as well because I lost all me friends and I don't go out anywhere, my partner does permanent nights and we only get together weekends, so most of the time I've got the grandson, so we don't get any time together, so on that eight week course it was lovely, really nice, I miss it, I do miss it.

Part of the work of the Partners for Protection programme is to educate mothers about abuse, the kind of person who commits it and how to keep a child safe. Where her own child has been abused and exhibits behaviours difficult to cope with, the course offers strategies to help a mother manage this and her child. The programme also offers space and time for participants to explore their own feelings and to help reduce feelings of isolation in the company of others in a similar situation.

As Carrie said:

> Just to talk to someone is like a mirror image of what had happened to me. Nobody had understood, nobody could.
>
> (Mosaic 2002)

This is one thing that makes the groups important: those who take part learn from each other. The most difficult thing about taking part is for participants to delve into their own childhoods. The most rewarding part of it is the opportunity to listen and support each other and not be frightened to be open and honest. Butler (2007) says that a great satisfaction felt by mothers is that, while knowing that there are "huge difficulties for you as a person, you can protect your child".

However, confronting such painful issues – one's own childhood, a probably broken relationship, the destruction of trust, what may have happened to one's child – is not without personal cost and has consequences for group dynamics. The conflicts we have with others can sometimes be because they arouse in us aspects of ourselves which we would prefer not to be there, to think about or to confront, or about which we are ambivalent, or they evoke in us the conflicted feelings we harbour about other people. The dynamics of the groups display all of this human drama, as Hill points out:

> Women still resident with abusive partners was a potential source of conflict. It was particularly conflictual for the woman herself, having to integrate information about their partner as an abuser, including his cycle [of abuse], elements of planning and deviant sexual arousal, and then returning home to him after the group. This was too difficult for one woman who dropped out of the group, the cognitive and emotional

distress too acute to tolerate. In attending the group she had been forced to confront the whole basis of their relationship: "My emotions towards [him] are swinging constantly. I feel I have been manipulated from day one. I wonder whether it's all been a sham ... I trusted him with my son. I tried to hard to protect my son and then invited the worst thing of all into my home. Did he ever want me?"

Group dynamics between women who wished to remain or rehabilitate with abusive partners and those who had made a decision to separate could have been provocative and destabilising, with such comments as "if he's abused Min [the woman's child], he still wouldn't be here, no way", and there was a risk of scapegoating of one woman who wanted her partner returned. However, this represented opposing sides of personal feelings expressed in all women: loathing and hatred versus a wish to forgive and focus on positive aspects of their partner and previous relationship. Where women were united was on self-blame, guilt and low self-worth, perceiving their children's abuse as a reflection of their worth both as women and mothers. Their self-doubts mirror those in society, despite our awareness that sexual abuse straddles all social [and] economic groups and is no respecter of intelligence, self-confidence or other attitudes people mistakenly identify as protective factors. These woman were not always within positions of disempowerment and abuse within relationships, rather they lacked the knowledge professionals have and without such knowledge were poorly equipped to deal with such a complex and challenging issue.

(Hill 2003: 6)

At the end of the course, the Partners for Protection programme offers each referring agency an assessment of the mother. This details their perceived capacity to protect their children in future, irrespective of whether or not they choose to be reunited with the partner who abused, although the assessment will take note of those women who do intend that.

However, Butler (2007) says:

If women come here to be reunited with their partners, we say that that is not what we are here for. It could be that the guy is too dangerous for that, in which case it's our job to help her to let go.

Of course, no one has the power to stop a woman making a decision to reunite with her partner, but if she does, then the children's services department will make a decision as to the likely safety of a child in the home and act accordingly.

It is not easy to monitor the effectiveness of the course in helping women to protect their children, because contact is not continued when the course comes to an end, other than if women choose to maintain in contact, as some do. However, says Butler (2007): "There is no way of unlearning what has been learned."

The value of the Partners for Protection programme is the creation of a safe space for the expression of conflict, self-doubt, disillusion, anger, disbelief and myriad other emotions which affect women whose partners have sexually abused children. It allows the creation of a woman's greater understanding and self-understanding so as to help her healing as a renewed individual who is also better equipped to protect her children.

Notes

A note on terminology

1 See Chapter 3, note 1.
2 The word "paedophile" is often taken generally to refer to someone who is sexually interested in pre-pubescent children, which itself says nothing about the age difference between the two parties. However, the somewhat loose definition and use of the term is contentious. This is partly because the word is commonly used to refer to those with a sexual interest in children, when the behaviours of child sex offenders are so varied. It is also taken to mean that those defined as such are sexually interested only in children. This ignores the many offenders who engage in sexual activity with children and adults (see Chapter 3). The association of the word with psychiatry can also imply that those who are "paedophiles" are in some way mentally abnormal by comparison with what are regarded as other norms of sexual behaviour.

I have found useful Cossins' definition of a sex offender. This is a "man or male adolescent who engages in contact or non-contact sexual activities with a child for the purposes of obtaining sexual gratification and who is: (i) at least five years older than the child; or (ii) younger, the same age as the child, or between one and four years older than the child in circumstances where the sexual activity was non-consensual". (A. Cossins, "Masculinities, sexualities and child sexual abuse", in G. Mair and R. Tarling (eds), *Papers from the British Society of Criminology Conference, Liverpool 1999*, British Society of Criminology, 2000).

Introduction

1 I am referring here to women who are married to or living with men who commit sexual offences against children who will often (but not always) be the woman's child or the child of the woman and her partner. Most of the women interviewed here had a child who was abused by their partner; the others joined the Partners for Protection programme because their partners had offended but not against their child. This book is not about those mothers of children who are abused but who are not married to, or living with the abuser as a partner.

1 Children, sexual abuse and its effects

1 For a description of the complicated family and other relationships which attach to many abused children and how they understand them see R. Rose, and T. Philpot, *The Child's Own Story: Life Story Work with Traumatised Children*, London: Jessica Kingsley Publishers (2005).

2 Local authority child protection registrations in England for sexual abuse declined from 2,700 in 2003 to 2,000 in 2007. Over the same period registrations for neglect rose from 10,600 to 12,500, as did emotional abuse, from 5,000 to 7,100. However, registrations for physical abuse fell from 4,300 to 3,500. *NSPCC Inform On-line Child Protection Resource*, www.nspcc.org.uk/inform.

3 When looking at ChildLine's statistics, it is wise to bear in mind that they refer not to the number of children and young people who contact the service but to the number of calls. So, for example, one child may make more than one call but, because ChildLine only records information that the child chooses to offer, exact statistics about individual children are difficult to come by. It also should be borne in mind that girls outnumber boys by a ratio of 4:1 in calling the service on almost any subject. This may skew the figures, but, given that females are more likely to report abuse than males and that more girls are abused than boys, it is likely that other estimates would indicate the same proportions.

2 A mother's lot

1 Ovaris (1991) expands, in some detail, on how Kubler-Ross's stages apply to non-offending mothers in the case of father–child incestuous relationships.

3 Child sex offenders and what we know about them

1 Grubin (1998) says that fewer than 5 per cent of sexual offences against children are known to be committed by women, often in association with men. However, population studies suggest that offending by women may be higher. This may be due to research by Bunting (2005), who suggests that professionals' lack of awareness and training may "hide" the figures.

2 It is worth noting that more than a third (36 per cent) of all rapes recorded by the police are committed against children under 16 years of age (Walker, Kershaw and Nicholas 2006). One source refers to "a broad consensus" that estimates that between 25 and 35 per cent of abusers are young people, mainly adolescent males (Lovell 2002). Home Office statistics show that 1.6 per cent of convictions and cautions in 2001 were of women (quoted in Stuart and Baines 2004).

3 Sanderson (2004) has very usefully tabulated Finkelhor's (1984) preconditions (table 3.1, pp. 94–5).

Graham Byers: "You can work through it"

1 The "risk swamp" is an exercise where each man on the offenders' course marks on a chart where he thinks he is in terms of high, medium or low risk of reoffending. The other men then give him feedback and, if he agrees, he will re-mark the chart to show a more realistic risk level. This is done at the start and the end of each block of the course as an indicator of the men's progress.

4 A place of safety

1 Since 1997 Mosaic's work has also been extended to take in group work with men serving sentences for offences against children. It is not known how many men it has worked with, but not all the men assessed go into a treatment group because they could be considered too low risk to need treatment; they lack motivation; or they have a personality disorder which does not make them susceptible to this kind of treatment. Also some matters, like dealing with sexual arousal, are not covered in a group but individually.

References

Anonymous (1994) "What has happened to us as a family after sexual abuse disclosure: A mother's story", *Child Care in Practice*, 1, 1: 14–15.

Bates, A., Saunders, R. and Wilson, C. (2007) "Doing something about it: A follow-up study of sex offenders participating in Thames Valley Circles of Support and Accountability", *British Journal of Community Justice*, 5, 1.

Beech, A., Erickson, M., Friendship, C. and Ditchfield, J. (2001) *A Six Year Follow-up of Men Going Through Probation-based Sex Offender Treatment Programmes*, Home Office Research Findings 144, London: Home Office.

Beech, A., Fisher, D., Beckett, R. and Scott-Fordham, A. (1998) *An Evaluation of the Prison Sex Offender Treatment Programme*, Home Office Research Findings No. 79, London: The Home Office.

Brickman, E., (1993) *Final Report: Child Sexual Abuse Public Policy Study*, New York: Victim Service.

Briggs, D., Doyle, P., Gooch, T. and Kennington, R. (1998) *Assessing Men Who Sexually Abuse. A Practice Guide*, London: Jessica Kingsley Publishers.

Brogden, M and Harkin, S. (2000) "Living with a convicted sex offender: Professional support for female partners", *Child Care in Practice*, 6, 1: January.

Bunting, L. (2005) *Females who Sexually Offend against Children: Responses of the Child Protection and Criminal Justice Systems*, London: NSPCC.

Butler, C. (2007) Interview with author. Unless otherwise stated all quotations in this chapter are based on interviews with the author.

Campbell, B. (1993) *Goliath: Britain's Dangerous Places*, London: Macmillan.

Cawson, P., Wattam, P., Brooker, S. and Kelly, G. (2000) *Child Maltreatment in the United Kingdom: A Study of the Prevalence of Child Abuse and Neglect*, London: NSPCC.

ChildLine (2003) *Annual Report*, London: ChildLine.

Clothier, H. (2008) *Partners for Protection Assessment Programme: Theory Manual*, Newcastle: The Sexual Behaviour Unit.

Condry, R. (2007) *Families Shamed: The Consequences of Crime for Relatives of Serious Offenders*, Cullompton: Willan Publishing.

Davies, J and Krane, J. (1996) "Shaking the legacy of mother blaming: No easy task for child welfare", *Journal of Progressive Human Services*, 7, 2: 3–22.

Deblinger, E., Stauffer, L. and Landsberg, C. (1994) "The impact of a history of child sexual abuse on maternal responses to allegations of sexual abuse concerning her child", *Journal of Sexual Abuse*, 3, 3: 67–75.

deMause, L. (1976) *The History of Childhood. Evolution and Parent–Child Relating as a Factor of History*, London: Souvenir Press.

deMause, L. (1991) "The universality of incest", *Journal of Psychotherapy*, 19, 2.

deMause, L. (1993) Paper presented to the British Psychological Society, London.

deMause, L. (1998) "The history of child abuse", *Journal of Psychotherapy*, 25, 3.

deMause, L., (2002) *The Emotional Life of Nations*, London: Karnac Books.

Department of Health (2003), *Safeguarding Children: What to Do if You are Worried a Child is Being Abused*. Children's Services Guidance. London: Department of Health.

Department of Health and the Home Office (2003) *The Victoria Climbe Inquiry. Report of an Inquiry*, London: The Stationery Office.

Department of Health and Social Security (1974), *Report of the Committee of Inquiry into the Care and Supervision Provided in Relation to Maria Colwell*. London: HMSO

Douglas, A. and Philpot, T. (1998) *Caring and Coping. A Guide to Social Services*, London: Routledge.

Egeland, B., Jacobvitz, D. and Stroufe, L.A. (1988) "Breaking the cycle of abuse", *Child Development*, 59: 1080–88.

Eldridge, H. (1998) *The Therapist's Guide for Maintaining Change: Relapse Prevention for Male Perpetrators of Child Sexual Abuse*, London: Sage.

Eldridge, H., Fuller, S., Findlater, D. and Palmer, T. (no date) *Helpline Report 2002–2005*, Alvechurch: Stop It Now!.

Everson, M.D., Hunter, W.M., Runyon, D.K., Edelsohn, G.A. and Coulter, M.L. (1989) "Maternal support following disclosure of incest", *American Journal of Orthopsychiatry*, 59, 2: 197–207.

Featherstone, B. and Evans, H. (2004) *Children Experiencing Maltreatment: Who do They Turn to?*, London: NSPCC.

Findlater, D. (2008) Private communication to author.

Finkelhor, D. (1984) *Child Sexual Abuse: New Theory and Research*, New York: Free Press.

Ford, H. and Beech, A. (2004a) *An Assessment of the Need for Residential Treatment Facilities for Child Sexual Offenders*, London: National Probation Service for England and Wales.

Ford, H. and Beech, A. (2004b) *The Effectiveness of the Wolvercote Clinic Residential Treatment Programme in Producing Short-term Treatment Changes and Reducing Sexual Reconvictions*, London: National Probation Service for England and Wales.

Glasser, M., Kolvin, I., Campbell, D., Glasser, A., Leitch, I. and Farrelly, S. (2001) "Cycle of child sexual abuse: Links between the victim and becoming a perpetrator", *British Journal of Psychiatry*, 179: 482–94.

Gomes-Schwarz, B., Horowitz, J.M. and Caldarelli, A.P. (1990) *Child Sexual Abuse. The Initial Effects*, California: Sage.

Goodwin, J. (1981) "Suicide attempts in sexual abuse victims and their mothers", *Child Abuse & Neglect*, 5: 217–21.

Grubin, D. (1998) *Sex Offending against Children: Understanding the Risk*, Police Research Series, paper 99, London: Home Office.

Guardian, The (2005) "Vital statistics: The world of women in numbers", 19 May.

Hanson, R.K., Gordon, A., Marques, J.K., Murphy., W and Quinsey, V.L. (2002) "First report of the collaborative outcome data project on the effectiveness of psychological treatment for sex offenders", *Sexual Abuse: Journal of Research & Treatment*, 14, 2: 169–94.

Hill, S. (2003) "Partners for Protection. A Possible Future Direction for Child Protection", Sexual Behaviour Unit/Mosaic, unpublished.

Home Office, H.M. Prison Service, National Probation Service for England and Wales (2002) *The Treatment and Risk Management of Sexual Offenders in Custody and in the Community*, London: Home Office.

Hooper, C.-A. (1992) *Mothers Surviving Child Sexual Abuse*, London; Routledge.

Hooper, C.-A. and Humphreys, C. (1998) "Women whose children have been sexually abused: Reflections on a debate" *British Journal of Social Work*, 28, 4: 565–80.

Humphreys, C. (1992) "Disclosure of child sexual assault: Implications for mothers", *Australian Social Work*, 45, 3: 27–35.

Humphreys, C. (1994) "Counteracting mother-blaming among child sexual abuse service providers: An experiential workshop", *Journal of Feminist Family Therapy*, 6, 1: 49–65.

Hunter, M. (2001) *Psychotherapy with Young People in Care: Lost and Found*, Hove: Brunner-Routledge.

Kelly, L., Regan, L and Burton, S. (1991) *An Exploratory Study of the Prevalence of Sexual Abuse in a Sample of 16–21 Year Olds*, London: Polytechnic of North London Sexual Abuse Studies Unit.

Kelley, S.J. (1990) "Responsibility and management strategies in child sexual abuse: A comparison of child protective workers, nurses and police officers", *Child Welfare*, 69, 1: 43–51.

Kempe, R. and Kempe, C. (1978) *Child Abuse*, London: Fontana/Open Books.

Kennington, R. (2008) Private communication to the author.

Kubler-Ross, E. (1970) *On Death and Dying*, London: Tavistock.

Lovell, E. (2002) *"I Think I Might Need Some Help with This Problem"*, London: NSPCC.

Mann, R.E. and Hollin, C.R. (2007) "Sexual offenders' explanations for their offending", *Journal of Sexual Aggression*, 13, 1: 3–9.

Mann, R.E., O'Brien, M., Thornton, D., Rallings, M., Webster, S. (2002) *Structured Assessment of Risk and* Need, London: H.M. Prison Department.

Marshall, P. (1997) *The Prevalence of Convictions for Sexual Offending*, Research Findings No. 55, London: Home Office.

Marshall, W.L., Barbaree, H.E. and Fernandez, Y. (1999) *Cognitive Behavioural Treatment of Sexual Offenders*, Chichester: Wiley.

Marshall, W.L., Fernandez, Y.M., Serran, G.A., Mulloy, R., Thornton, D., Mann, R.E. and Anderson, D. (2003) "Process variables in the treatment of sexual offenders. A review of the relevant literature", *Journal of Aggression and Violent Behaviour*, 8: 205–34.

Massat, C.R. and Lundy, M. (1998) "'Reporting costs to non-offending parents in cases of intrafamilial child sexual abuse", *Child Welfare*, 78, 4: 371–88.

Moore, J. (1992) *The ABC of Child Protection*, Aldershot: Ashgate.

Morrison, N.C. and Clavenna-Valleroy, J. (1998) "Perceptions of material support and treatment outcomes in sexually abused female adolescents", *Journal of Child Sexual Abuse*, 7: 23–40.

Mosaic (2002) Interview on video made for internal use.

Mosaic Women Writers' Group (no date) *Picking up the Pieces: A Collection of Poetry and Writings*, Newcastle: Barnardo's Mosaic Project.

Mudaly, N. and Goddard, C. (2006) *The Truth is Longer than a Lie: Children's Experience of Abuse and Professional Interventions*, London: Jessica Kingsley Publishing.

Myer, M.H. (1985) "A new look at mothers of incest victims", *Journal of Social Work and Human Sexuality*, 3: 47–58.

Ovaris, W. (1991) *After the Nightmare. The Treatment of Non-Offending Mothers of Sexually Abused Children*, Holmes Beach, FL: Learning Publications

Pellegrin, A. and Wagner, W.G. (1990) "Child sexual abuse: Factors affecting victims' removal from home", *Child Abuse & Neglect*, 14: 53–60.

Philpot, T. (1994) *Action for Children: The Story of Britain's Foremost Children's Charity*, Oxford: Lion Publishing.

Plotnikoff, J and Wolfson, R. (2005) *In their Own Words: The Experiences of 50 Young Witnesses in Criminal Proceedings*, London: NSPCC.

Plummer, C.A. (2006) "The discovery process: What mothers see and do in gaining awareness of the sexual abuse of their children", *Child Abuse & Neglect*, 30, 11: 1227–37.

Pughe, B. and Philpot, T. (2007) *Living Alongside the Child's Recovery: Therapeutic Parenting with Traumatised Children*, London and Philadelphia: Jessica Kingsley Publishers.

Reid, C. (1989) *Mothers of Sexually Abused Girls: A Feminist View*, Norwich: Social Work Monographs, University of East Anglia.

Rose, J. (1987) *For the Sake of the Children: Inside Barnardo's: 120 Years of Caring for Children*, London: Hodder & Stoughton.

Rymaszewska, J. and Philpot, T. (2006) *Reaching the Vulnerable Child: Therapy with Traumatized Children*, London: Jessica Kingsley Publishers.

Salter, A. (2003) *Predators, Paedophiles, Rapists and other Sex Offenders: Who They Are, How They Operate and How We Can Protect Ourselves and Our Children*, New York: Basic Books.

Sanderson, C. (2004) *The Seduction of Children. Empowering Parents and Teachers to Protect Children from Child Sexual Abuse*, London: Jessica Kingsley Publishers.

Silverman, J. and Wilson, D. (2002) *Innocence Betrayed: Paedophilia, the Media and Society*, Cambridge: Polity Press.

Sirles, Elizabeth, A. and Franke, Pamela J. (1989) "Factors influencing mothers' reactions to intrafamily sexual abuse", *Child Abuse & Neglect*, 13: 131–39.

Skuse, D. (2003) quoted in *The Guardian*, quoted by Sanderson, C. (2004) *The Seduction of Children. Empowering Parents and Teachers to Protect Children from Child Sexual Abuse*, London: Jessica Kingsley Publishers.

Smith, G. (1994), "Parent, partner, protector: Conflicting role demands for mothers of sexually abused children", in Morrison, T., Erooga, M. and Beckett, R.C. (eds), *Sexual Offending against Children: Assessment and Treatment of Male Abusers*. London: Routledge.

Stuart, M. and Baines, C. (2004) *Safeguards for Vulnerable Children: Three Studies on Abusers, Disabled Children and Children in Prison*, York: Joseph Rowntree Foundation.

Wagner, William G. (1991) "Depression in mothers of sexually abused vs mothers of nonabused children", *Child Abuse & Neglect*, 15: 99–104.

Walker, A., Kershaw, C. and Nicholas, S. (2006) *Crime in England Wales 2005–6*, London: Home Office.

Walsh, P. (no date) "Therapeutic strategies for sex offenders: Contents and rationale", unpublished paper.

Wattam, C and Woodward, C. (1996) "'And do I abuse my children? No!' Learning about prevention from people who have experienced child abuse", *Childhood Matters*, vol. 2, London: HMSO.

Wilson, R.J., Picheca, J.E. and Prinzo, M. (2007) "Evaluating the effectiveness of professionally-facilitated volunteerism in the community-based management of high-risk sexual offenders: part two – a comparison of recidivism rates", *Howard Journal of Criminal Justice*, 46, 4: 327–37.

Wolf, S.C., (1984) "A multifactor model of defiant sexuality", paper presented at Third International Conference on Victimology, Lisbon, Portugal, November, quoted in Sanderson, C. (2004) *The Seduction of Children: Empowering Parents and Teachers to Protect Child from Child Sexual Abuse*. London: Jessica Kingsley Publishers.

Wyre, R. (2004) quoted in Sanderson, C., *The Seduction of Children: Empowering Parents and Teachers to Protect Children against Child Sexual Abuse*, London: Jessica Kingsley Publishers.

Wyre, R. (2007) Talk on the partners of sex offenders, Community Care Live, London, 11 October.